10 YEARS
YOUNGER

10 YEARS YOUNGER

21 SURPRISING TECHNIQUES TO TURN BACK TIME

By

KYLIE ANSETT Medical Herbalist

Disclaimer

This book is not meant to replace or undermine a face to face consultation with a health care provider. Its purpose is to empower you to take your health and healing into your own hands, to get to know your body and to start to listen to it.

Dedication

To my son, Dylan.
You have kept me young!
I admire your spirit so much.

For more information please email: kylie@kylieansett.com

ISBN: 1535225378
ISBN-13: 978-1535225373
ASIN: B01F262842

Contents

Disclaimer..iv

Dedication...v

Acknowledgements...ix

Preface..xi

Made you look 3

Who am I?...5

Are You Up for The Challenge? 7

The Truth about Youth 11

SKIN 13

Chapter 1: The Power of Sour.............................15

Chapter 2: The Ancient Science of the Skin 19

Chapter 3: Can You Brush Your Liver?..............23

FACE 27

Chapter 4: What if Your Face could go to the Gym?........29

Chapter 5: Can You Rub Out Wrinkles? 33

Chapter 6: The Spectacle Conspiracy 37

Chapter 7: The Silent Treatment Everyone is
Talking About 43

BODY 47

    Chapter 8: What Cats Know 49

    Chapter 9: In Defence of the Womb 53

    Chapter 10: What Plants Eat 59

    Chapter 11: Do Shoes Make You Old? 63

    Chapter 12: Twenty-five Thousand Times a Day 67

    Chapter 13: Green is the New Black 71

    Chapter 14: Take with a Pinch of Salt 77

    Chapter 15: (Almost) Better than Sex 81

    Chapter 16: Where We All Came From 85

MIND 89

    Chapter 17: Why this Daily Routine Ages You 91

    Chapter 18: The Power of Dark 97

    Chapter 19: Words Change Everything 103

    Chapter 20: How to Stack the Deck 107

    Chapter 21: Put Your Doctor Out of Business 113

    Chapter 22: Putting it All Together 117

    Chapter 23: Attitude 121

    Chapter 24: Special Mentions 125

    Chapter 25: Things to Avoid 129

    Chapter 26: Confession 135

Note on Index of Ailments 137

Index of Ailments 139

A gift for you... Infographic of the Book 153

About the Author 155

Acknowledgements

It is always a pleasure to put your head up at the end of the lengthy process of writing a book and see so many people cheering you on. I would like to acknowledge several people specifically, but foremost in my mind is my mentor Elaine Hollingsworth who inspired me to take control of my health way back when. Her influence has changed the course of my life. It has enabled me to empower my clients, which is a gift and my greatest joy. I am indebted to my coach Kevin Bees who so skillfully challenged me. My writing buddy Cindy Kennedy who encourages, inspires and keeps me on track. My mastermind group who uplift me. I am forever grateful for the support and encouragement of my family and friends which humbles me.

Thank you all.

Preface

The 21 techniques in the following pages as well as the special mentions have all been tried and tested by myself and by hundreds of my clients over the course of fifteen years as a practitioner.

My area of expertise is health, not disease. I leave the study and treatment of that to the disease industry. But as almost all illnesses can be cured by robust mental, physical and emotional health, it is a natural conclusion to draw that the answer to your disease does not lie in medications, operation and that make you unwell. However. I will let you draw your own conclusion.

10 Years Younger promises to make you feel and look younger and healthier, fitter and happier. Big declarations, I know, but my challenge to you is to put them to the test and see for yourself.

10 YEARS
YOUNGER

Made you look

There is no way around it. You are getting older. You want to look younger because our culture tells you a million times a day, in a million subtle (and not so subtle) ways that you have to. We have *all* bought into it. This obsession with youth has spawned a billion dollar industry. And kept women of wisdom from stepping up. After all, it's hard to succeed at world domination if you are busy worrying about your wrinkles and your waistline.

We live in a culture that worships youth and despises age. Unlike many native cultures which respect and deeply value their elders, we do neither. But like it or not, every one of us is aging. Constantly and continuously. Until we die.

This book is not another tool to play into this cultural delusion. This book is about claiming your power. Here you will find alternatives to chemical, surgical and artificial procedures that are designed to erode your confidence and empty your wallet. Along the way you will uncover a vibrant, powerful and youthful self within.

I encourage you to embrace who you are and where your body is at. Age is a state of mind with very little to do with when we were born. If you follow even just some of these routines, you will notice a difference in how you feel and very soon, in how you look.

Looking and feeling ten years younger *is* possible. This book contains the secrets to the elixir of youth.

Who am I?

So who am I to talk about looking and feeling ten years younger?

Apparently I don't look (or act) my age. So I guess that gives me some sort of authority on the topic. I am often mistaken for being far younger than I am. Many people flat out refuse to believe I have an adult son. I'm forty-eight, you know, that age in our culture, when it is supposedly it is all over for a woman. I have no issue with being the age I am or with looking my age. I am, however, all about how I feel.

The techniques in this book are a collection of my favourite youth elixirs. They have helped keep me looking ten years younger, but more importantly, way more importantly, they make me *feel* ten years younger.

I have been a holistic health and alternative medical practitioner for over twenty years. My greatest passion is to help my patients uncover their inner health. I want them to be able to trust their own bodies, I want to empower them to be in charge of their health.

So, I have made a study of well-being. Of feeling good. Of true health. And I see health as not just the absence of disease. True health is the life-giving, energy-producing, endorphin-making vigour we associate with youth. It has become my passion. My obsession. My calling. I have looked deep into thousands of eyes as an iridologist. I have palpated millions of muscles as a bodyworker. And I have raved about green smoothies to more people than I could count. I feel I have a handle on wellbeing. On health. Maybe even on that secret elixir of youth.

Are You Up for
The Challenge?

We'd all love to not only look but *feel* younger. Getting older, after all, doesn't feel that good. Loss of energy. Diminishing senses. Fading looks. It's not exactly *fun*. But does it *have* to be this way? Is boundless energy and fresh-faced optimism the exclusive right of the young? After all, I know twenty year olds who drag the weight of the world around. Who look and act decades older. And I know women in their seventies who energise every conversation. Whose open-mindedness and vigour makes them appear far younger than they are. I am sure you do too.

We are all searching for the secret formula. We all want to feel like the energetic, open-minded fresh-faced self that we were ten, twenty years ago. We'd also like the wisdom we have earned to get there, only without the wrinkles that go with it.

This book will show you twenty-one techniques to keep you looking and feeling young. I guarantee that along with a few you may expect to see, you will find some surprising and unusual techniques you have probably never heard of before.

I have gathered together twenty-one of the best techniques (plus a couple of bonuses!) that have worked for me and many of my patients. They are all easy to do so you will see results fast.

This book will take you down the path to a younger, more vibrant you. From white teeth to firm skin. From sweet breath to a happier vagina. Forget dangerous surgery. Forget expensive chemicals. Simple. Inexpensive. Immediate. Actionable. I will show you the *how*, while appealing to your intelligence and explaining the *why*.

But with all, I encourage you to do your own research. To make sure they are right for *you*. For *your* body. You are the expert on that. I am simply showing you the methods.

So here is the challenge: choose a technique a day and put it into action. Do this for the next seven days. The next week keep a couple you love and want to continue doing and add seven more. For the last week continue doing three favorites from the last fortnight and add the final seven.

After twenty-one days you will have tried all the methods and you can create a program that is suited to both your body and your lifestyle. One that you can easily integrate into your life and keep up.

There is no need (and no time!) to do all techniques every day. At different times of your life you will need some more than others. Some you will love and find so useful you will immediately keep forever. Others will not suit you at all. But try them all out so you know what

To make it easier for you I have created a schedule. I have divided the twenty-one techniques into the time they take, the ease to perform, the part of the body they act upon and the way they act. You can access the challenge schedule at this link: https://app.convertkit.com/landing_pages/46867

Following this plan you can start simple and gradually get more complex. The download includes a mock copy and a few blank sheets that you can print out and fill in with your own schedule.

The idea is to make it work *for you!*

The Truth about Youth

One day, two men in neat, dark suits came down our driveway. We lived on a five-acre property with a long driveway. My son and I were out the front of the house at the time, deep in conversation. As they rounded the final bend, they greeted us, real estate flyers in hand, and asked: "Are your parents home?" Apparently to the local property hawkers I was lumped in with my lanky seventeen-year-old. I answered them, "Ummm…well *his* are, but not *mine*." I was almost forty at the time.

Quick Quiz. Did they think I was the sister / friend because of:

1. The way I looked
2. My attitude

I think it was attitude. I am not wrinkle free, toned or taut. I think the energy I gave off, we were both lounging on the bonnet of my car, had more to do with their mistaken identity than anything else.

And this was not an isolated incident. In his late teens my son was taken by his friends to the hospital with a broken collar bone after a bike accident. When I arrived to see him I was told I had to wait until his 'parents' arrived.

I don't know if all of this makes me an authority. But I have a few tricks up my sleeve. Some will be revolutionary. Will make you reassess the way you have been doing things for ever. Will give you alternatives that are easy to implement. Cost efficient. Quick to do. And that help you not only look at least ten years younger, but far more importantly, feel it.

My formula is:

- ☐ Simple
- ☐ Cheap
- ☐ Fast
- ☐ Effective

Let's dive in!

SKIN

Your skin is about what is going on inside, not what you apply to the outside

CHAPTER I

The Power of Sour

This technique is not for the weak-bladdered traveller. I made the mistake of drenching before an hour long car trip. There was a lot of leg crossing and seat wiggling near the end and when I arrived I had to double park my car and make a beeline for the bathrooms.

However, if you have the luxury of having access to a toilet in the first hour of your day, this is the *best* thing to do for your liver. And boy, does your poor liver need all the help it can get.

Warm lemon juice has an amazing effect on the whole body. The digestive system. The immune system. The bowel. It will lower your blood pressure and help you lose weight. I have had patients reverse a fatty liver doing nothing more than this. Here's something that might surprise you: lemons, those most acidic of fruit, *alkalises* your whole system.

So how does warm lemon juice make you younger? Your liver is the major detoxifier of the body. It filters out the pollution, chemicals and pesticides that you breathe, eat, drink and even think (yes, you can think yourself old or young, see chapter twenty-one for more on that).

Living the modern life we do, our livers are working pretty hard all day, every day, just to get by. When the liver is overloaded it will pass off some of the detoxifying work to your skin. Hives. Itchiness. Dry or oily. Odorous. Discoloured. Dull. Your skin will be less vibrant as it struggles with a toxic backlog. You will look and feel older. And squeezing out, scraping off, covering up or ointmenting over doesn't help much either. Those pimples? That rash? It's the crap on the inside trying to get out. Treating bad skin caused by liver overload with supressing medications (like cortisone), is like painting over dry rot in the basement and saying "Look! All better!" Most likely the rot will come bubbling through the paint in a matter of weeks, but the really scary thing is when your kitchen floor collapses one night. Yeah, that is when after years of covering up, suppressing and ignoring the small cries for help your body has been giving you, it finally throws up an insidious, incurable, chronic auto-immune disorder, a mental imbalance or worse. How do *you* think cancer starts?

Reflux, arthritis or gout? Get into the warm lemon drenching (maybe start with a teaspoon of juice, not a litre, if you have reflux). The fruit has a lot of acidity, but as it is processed by the body it creates an alkaline environment. So if you want to alkalise (and who doesn't – more on the amazing benefits of that in chapter thirteen) drenching with lemon is the way to go.

Support your liver and you will feel a million bucks. Your bowel will be eliminating with ease (see chapter fifteen for the low down on elimination). Your skin will start to glow as the liver performs its job with ease. There will be a skip in your step as you move lighter and brighter through your day. If you have a lemon tree it won't even cost you anything. If you don't have one, make friends with someone who does. Or plant one now.

~ EXERCISE ~

Lemon Drench

I call this Lemon Drench because the idea is to infuse all of your cells. Saturate your system. Drench.

TIME: Half an hour.

FREQUENCY: Daily. Nice to do whilst stretching.

TOOLS: Lemons, warm water

METHOD: First thing in the morning. Squeeze a lemon into a jug of warm water and drink over the next 1/2 hour. Give your teeth a rinse with fresh water when finished to protect the enamel. Start with a quarter of a lemon and work up to one lemon in one litre (two pints) of warm water. If your bowels 'react', start with just a teaspoon of lemon for a few weeks until your system gets used to it.

Ticks all the boxes!

▶ Simple ✓   ▶ Cheap ✓   ▶ Fast ✓   ▶ Effective ✓

CHAPTER 2

———•———

The Ancient Science
of the Skin

Having toned radiant skin is an outward sign of youth and vitality. It looks amazing. It feels even better.

The first time I did this my bathroom looked like a pipe had burst. As I staggered from hot bath to icy shower the floor was drenched. The first few rounds were painful. I thought I would pass out from the heat. Then the cold was unbearable. Painful! But after the third round something strange happened. I think my body gave up resisting.

Hydrotherapy is nothing new. The Romans and Greeks were big on it. Even the Egyptians and Persians were aficionados. The Japanese made an art form of it. And in the late nineteenth century the Europeans and British discovered and embraced it. It was all the rage to convalesce at a Hydrotherapy resort in a sunny location if you were diagnosed with consumption. Or alcoholism. Or the sniffles. Or pretty much anything. I think it may have been more about the getting away than anything else. It has been practiced for centuries.

A monthly hot/cold session will make you feel like you have had ten massages. I'm not kidding. This is one to do at the end of the day and then curl up into bed.

~ EXERCISE ~

Hot/Cold Water Therapy

TIME: 20-30 mins

FREQUENCY: 1 x month

TOOLS:

- A separate bath and shower (but in the same room).
- A heap of towels/bathmats.
- Plenty of hot water.
- Bath salts are an optional extra.
- Run the bath and make it hot. I mean scalding. Like thirty-nine degrees C (102 F). Just a bit hotter than you would be comfortable with.
- Have a trail of towels or bath mats on the floor between the bath and shower. Depending on how much hot water you have available you may need to use a kettle. Have it plugged in somewhere that it can be easily accessed.

METHOD:

- Wash yourself briefly first in the shower (to keep the bath clean).
- A dry body brush session (see chapter three) beforehand would be ideal.

- Immerse yourself in the bath for as long as you are able. It may only be a few minutes.
- Then go straight to the cold shower. Don't be a wuss. For as long as you can stand. Which may be only thirty seconds. That's fine.
- Then it's back into the piping hot bath.
- Repeat. At least five rounds.

Keep the bath water hot by topping up as needed (my hot water always runs out, hence the kettle).

After a round or two, you will find you are able to extend the time of each round. After the third round you won't even notice how cold the shower is. By the fifth your body simply gives up. Turns to mush.

Caution: use your good sense. Only do this if you are feeling robust. Do not do if you are pregnant or extremely weak or unwell. You may like to have a buddy nearby: all that water can get slippery. If you don't think you are quite up to it, you can tone down the heat and the cold. You're in charge. Take responsibility. I'm just telling what I do. But if I felt faint or lightheaded I would be super cautious. You probably should too.

▶ Simple ✓   ▶ Cheap ✓   ▶ Effective ✓

CHAPTER 3

Can You Brush Your Liver?

Smooth flawless skin is the holy grail of youthful vitality. It is enticing to touch. Radiant to see. Intoxicating to smell. Youthful skin is a direct reflection of what is going on inside of you. A clear message from your body. How can you get and maintain radiant, youthful skin?

It might surprise you to know that, as well as the bowel and bladder, you also eliminate through your skin. A well-functioning body will use the massive surface area of the skin of our entire body to remove toxins and waste. It goes via the liver (which filters all toxins) to the surface of our skin and is got rid of in the form of dead skin cells and sweat.

If our skin is not eliminating effectively this dead toxic layer sits just beneath the surface making our skin dull and lifeless. Rough, dry or oily. Blotchy. We get pimples and blemishes. Hives and rashes. We become more prone to asthma and allergies.

Modern living exposes us to a constant load of toxins. The air we breathe. The food we eat. The water we drink. It's not to say they are *poisonous* but there are chemicals and pollutants in our air, food and water that our liver constantly has to filter.

And we don't make the job of elimination any easier for our skin. We are covered up much of the time. Often with synthetic clothing. We use soap, which clogs pores. We lather on creams and lotions and perfumes which further block things. The worst is antiperspirant, which is so counter intuitive (more on that particular aging habit in chapter fourteen). All this inhibits the skins natural detoxification, its ability to 'breathe'.

The famous nineteenth century naturopath, Dr. Bernard Jenson, the founder of modern iridology, was a great supporter of dry body brushing. He believed that many patients' problems could be traced back to a burdened liver, crippled under a toxic load of chemicals and pollution. And the skin, instead of helping the detoxification process, was inert. This symptom is seen in the iris as a *scurf rim*: a dark circular ring at the outer edge of the iris. If you had this sign the diagnosis was that your skin was poorly eliminating.

Daily dry body brushing allows the skin to *breathe*. Finally, that load of dead cells is removed, revealing fresh, clear and youthful skin beneath. And you don't even have to go to the salon for an expensive, toxic chemical peel.

You may think dry body brushing is the same as using a loofah or exfoliating. It is not! It is quite different. You do it dry. It allows a much more vigorous removal of cells.

Dr. Jenson recommended *dry body brushing* to treat this frequently seen symptom. However, he was frustrated at the lack of quality tools available to do the job effectively. So he created a quality brush for the job. It has a long, detachable handle. It has extra-long, robust bristles made from Tampico (a natural fibre). Today these are still the best brushes for this task. You can also get long-handled body brushes from most reputable health food stores. Just make sure they have *natural* bristles (not nylon).

~ EXERCISE ~

Dry Body Brushing
___

TIME: 5 mins

FREQUENCY: Daily

TOOLS: Long-handled, natural bristle brush

METHOD:

- Start dry, before you shower.
- Be vigorous.
- Begin at the soles of your feet & work toward the heart.
- Use a circular motion.
- Avoid delicate areas (face, breasts).
- Give extra attention to rough skin (elbows, heels, scars)
- Spend extra time on cellulite (thighs, buttocks).

Care of your brush: 'Clean' by placing in sunlight for a few hours. Do not clean with water – it will lose its robust texture. Replace as you would a tooth brush, when it starts to wear, or become too soft, around every six to nine months.

Ticks all the boxes!

▶ Simple ✓   ▶ Cheap ✓   ▶ Fast ✓   ▶ Effective ✓

FACE

Your face is your business card to the world

CHAPTER 4

What if Your Face could go to the Gym?

My brother made a video of himself shaving in the mirror. He stretched his face this way and that to get the razor across every contour, nook and cranny. It made me think - have you ever noticed, that despite all the expensive age defying creams and lotions women use, many men's facial skin ages slower than women's?

We all know all about exercising to help tone the muscles of your body. Well your face is made up of many tiny muscles. They may be small, but they are no less significant. No less in need to stretching to keep them happy and firm. Just as responsive to toning exercises to reduce sagging skin and prevent wrinkles forming.

~ EXERCISE ~

Face Gym

You can do face stretching whenever, wherever. It's a great time killer at traffic lights when in the car. I get some strange looks, but that is all part of the fun! I draw the line at doing it at the queue at the bank though.

TIME: 10 mins can be broken up into several smaller sessions

FREQUENCY: Daily

TOOLS: Your face

METHOD:

- Smile/Kiss 10 x
    - Do a big smile. Grin from ear to ear. Really stretch it out. Try and reach each ear with the corners of your mouth
    - Then bring the corners right in to a kissy purse, one where you are really squeezing your lips out as far as they will go
    - Then back to the grin
    - Then back to the purse
- Yawn/Kiss 10 x
    - Make the biggest O that you can with your mouth
    - Then bring it back to a kissy purse

- o Then back
- o And forth

- Yawn/tongue 10 x
  - o Do a big O again but this time stick your tongue out as far as you can at the same time
  - o Relax
  - o Back to the tongue

- Eyebrow raise 10 x
  - o Elevate just your eyebrows
  - o Hold for a few seconds
  - o Relax
  - o Make sure to keep your eyes neutral
  - o Really feel the skin between your brows stretching

- Surprised eyes 10 x
  - o Open your eyes as wide as possible
  - o Hold for a few seconds
  - o Relax
  - o Repeat

- Squinty eyes 10 x
  - o Raise the lower lid of your eyes
  - o Keep the eyes open
  - o Hold for a few seconds
  - o Relax
  - o Repeat

- Neck grimace 10 x
  - o Make a grimace with your lower mouth
  - o This will cause the neck to stretch
  - o Hold for a few seconds
  - o Repeat

Doesn't that feel amazing? You can go to town on all areas of your face. The trick is repetition. And building the reps slowly over time. Just like you would doing any type of exercise.

▶ Simple ✓   ▶ Cheap ✓   ▶ Effective ✓

CHAPTER 5

Can You Rub Out Wrinkles?

Forget about chemical peels, Botox or even facelifts. Your face is made up of forty-three muscles. They are constantly working. Frowning, smiling, being surprised. Snickering. Grimacing. And we all have our favourite 'go-to' expressions, don't we? After a while it shows. Repeatedly used expressions start to wear a little track in our face. Then a deeper one. After a certain age you can know a person by their face.

I hope you enjoyed ironing out your wrinkles by doing face gym in chapter four, but you may be surprised to know that toxins can also get locked into those tiny muscles. Nutrient laden oxygen is not circulating bringing revitalising properties. It causes your skin to look dull and lifeless. To be prone to blemishes and uneven pigmentation.

Precise Point Massage not only releases bound in toxins but also brings fresh nutrient-laded oxygen to the right areas. This inhibits the production of collagen destroying free radicals. Far more effective than expensive pots of designer creams. A ten-minute treatment will take years off a tired face. Immediately.

I love doing this for my clients when they get a body treatment. They swear it takes years off *immediately*!

So, the answer to the question: Can you rub out wrinkles? Is: "Yes!" and here's how…

~ EXERCISE ~

Precise Point Massage

TIME: 10 mins

FREQUENCY: 1 x weekly

TOOLS: Have a clean make up free face and short nails.

METHOD: Work the hot spots: The forehead. The eyebrows. The hairline. The cheekbones. The chin. It may be tender, that's okay. What you are feeling are the locked in toxins. As you spend more time on an area the pain will dissipate.

General rules: As deep as you can bear. Chase the pain. Use circles, figure eights, up and down and back and forth.

- Between the eyebrows
  - o Use flat or side of knuckles
  - o Right into hairline
  - o Move along under the brow ridge

- Eyebrows
  - o Use finger tips or flat of knuckles
  - o Work along them right to the ends
  - o Go under the ridge
  - o Tiny circular movements

- Forehead

- o Use the flat of your lower finger joint
- o Include scalp line
- o Include temples

- Cheekbones
  - o Fingertips
  - o Gentler pressure
  - o Along the whole ridge
  - o Find the spot near the nose where the cheek flesh begins
  - o Find the tender points and focus in on them

- Chin
  - o Finger tips
  - o Circular motion
  - o Work really deeply

- Ears
  - o Vigorous and over entire ear
  - o Squeeze and pinch
  - o Top to bottom and back again

Toxins are released into the lymph and blood stream to be eliminated in your waste. So drink lots of fresh water after this process.

► Simple ✓   ► Cheap ✓   ► Effective ✓

CHAPTER 6

The Spectacle Conspiracy

Most people just accept that as we get older we will need glasses. It is a given. But what if it was not? What if the *need* for glasses was as manufactured as the product? And what if you could reverse the vision challenges that so often come with age?

What if glasses were just a crutch? There appears to be an optometrist on every corner now and they are a hungry industry. When vision starts to fade, we line up to get our free eye test and are told we will need glasses for the rest of our lives. Every year the prescription gets stronger and stronger. It is accepted. So we do it.

So how can *you* buck the system? Be the exception? I started to need to enlarge many of the things I was reading on screen. I got rather annoyed with technicians who asked me to read the black on black, six-point numerals on faulty devices. A joke I was finding less and less funny. Then I discovered that the reason my eyes were not seeing so sharply was more to do with my muscles than anything else.

I think we imagine our eyes getting elderly along with the rest of our body and just not working any more. Well, your eyes work. But to focus they rely on tiny muscles that maneuverer them. Like a puppet is moved by its strings. There are tiny little string-like muscles at the top, bottom and sides of your eye balls. And what do these tiny muscles do? They change the shape of your pupil, allowing you to focus.

Have you ever felt the muscles at the back of your neck after a stressful day? Or your scalp muscles? Tight and hard right? So how does your scalp get tight?

Well it's called stress. That old chestnut that is the bane of modern living. And stress does not have to mean you are going through a divorce, moving house or have lost a loved one. Simply being alive is stressful. Dealing with alarm clocks, tardy children, rushing through traffic, a judgemental look from your neighbour when you haven't cut the grass. Not to mention the more obvious stress inducers like an argument with a spouse, illness or work problems. But to your body, even things like going to the gym are experienced as stress. So yeah, it's everywhere, its constant and we all suffer from its effects.

So what has stress to do with your eyes?

Well like tightness in your neck muscles, stress will also tighten those tiny eye muscles. Were you ever able to do the splits? Okay, well, how about touching our toes? Can you still do it now? If you don't stretch regularly, the answer is probably no.

But if you *started* stretching you would soon be reaching your toes. Those tiny eye muscle also need to stretch and contract with ease to effectively convex or concave your pupil and allow you to see clearly. If they are stiff, like your neck, or rusty like your hamstrings, or inactive like your abs, they will not be able to perform their job well.

The problem with glasses is that they train your eyes muscles to be lazy. So if they were working at eighty percent capacity, after a few years with glasses, they will be at seventy percent. Then sixty. With inactivity they get lazy, tight and immobile.

You may never be able to do the splits again, but with simple exercise you can regain some of the flexibility that allows you to see naturally. Without glasses.

So how do you release tight eye muscles? It's simple and it's fun!

~ EXERCISE ~

Natural Vision Exercises

TIME: 1-2 mins on each exercise

FREQUENCY: Daily

TOOLS: Your eyes!

METHOD:

Here are 4 easy exercises for your eye health. Sunning, Palming, Pencil Nose and Near/Far.

1. *Sunning* is relaxing and beautiful. You *need* sunlight for good eye health (Go to chapter ten to see why), but now you're going to sit in the sun with your eyes closed for a few minutes. Allow the sunlight to softly absorb through your eyelids. No burning (be sensible). Tiny amounts of sunlight, with all its healing properties are absorbed through the eyelids. (See chapter ten for more information on the danger of sunglasses)

2. *Palming* is great to do during or after a stressful day. Sit at a table. Vigorously rub your palms together for a few minutes to create heat with the friction. With eyes closed, cup your warm palms over each eye socket. Lean forward, resting your elbows on the table or a cushion.

Breath. Feel the warmth, the darkness. Let your eyes absorb the heat. Let your eyes relax.

3. *Near/Far* is the perfect exercise to work out and stretch those tiny eye muscles. Especially when they have been focused at one distance for long periods. Like when you have been staring at a screen. Which I'm guessing we are all guilty of from time to time. It creates RSI of the eyes. Our beautiful eyes are meant to focus on many different distances throughout the day. If you were in nature, you would look at the ground, then at the mountain tops, then the horizon, then the bark of a tree. You may pause to examine a tiny insect, spot a bird in the tree tops, scan the clouds for rain. Constantly your eyes are flicking between dozens of different distances. Near/Far. Far/near.

Each time your eye muscles are stretching, contracting, elongating, shortening. Moving! Keeping supple and flexible. RSI is caused when you repeatedly move a muscle in a small range. So staring at the computer screen keeps the focus at the same distance for hours upon hours. The muscles become stiff from lack of use.

After a while (years) they start to calcify in that shortened state. Then when you want to use them they are non-responsive. And so it's off to the optometrist and the spectacle merry-go-round begins.

At regular times through the day take a few minutes to focus on different distances. Simply take your eyes away from the screen and look out the window, at the horizon, at your knee, at the grass or road or rooftops, at the sky etc. Near/far, far/near. Really far, really near. Back and forth. Soften and flex those tight tired muscles. Use a soft, unfocussed and fluid movement.

4. *Pencil Nose* is great to stimulate tired eyes. Imagine you have a pencil on the end of your nose. Now 'draw' an outline around everything you can see. The picture frame, the window, the tree, your desk, the cup. The idea is to not just move your eyes, but your whole head. It creates a relaxing rhythm. After a few minute of doing this the muscles soften and relax.

Ticks all the boxes!

► Simple ✓   ► Cheap ✓   ► Fast ✓   ► Effective ✓

CHAPTER 7

The Silent Treatment Everyone is Talking About

We all want lovely, white teeth. And sweet breath. But what about waking with a clean feeling in your mouth instead of that 'bottom of the budgie's cage' taste? What if you could cure (mild) toothache? Bleeding gums? Gingivitis (inflamed gums). What if you could put your dentist out of work? It's not like he needs another trip to Aspen this year, is it? If you look and smell that sweet, there must be something good going.

Oil pulling is an ancient Ayurvedic therapy. It involves oil. And your mouth. And about five to twenty minutes of silence. That's right. No talking! For some this is the real challenge of this task. I have tried to answer the phone whilst doing this treatment. I had my head tilted back and it sounded like I was underwater. They were asking me "What? Where ARE you? Are you okay?"

You see, I used to drink a lot of tea. Six, seven cups a day. All that tannin takes its toll. Stained teeth are nasty. It's not like it was tobacco-chewing, hillbilly bad; just not quite white. And chemical whitening scares me; all those chemicals! Not to mention there is something cartoonish about the blinding, Hollywood smirk.

And then I discovered oil pulling. Those ancient Indians knew a thing or two about tea drinking, after all. Simple. Minutes a day. White teeth. Not only that but sooo many more benefits. Benefits for longevity and inner youthfulness. So now it's part of my daily routine.

You may like to turn this into a family routine. Twenty minutes before leaving, everyone takes a mouthful of oil, then as you exit, you all spit. Calmly, happily... *silently*! It will revolutionise the morning rush.

The mouth is a natural repository for bacteria. The body employs many different methods to eliminate. The skin. The mouth, the saliva, the blood. The breath is another major method of elimination. Every time we exhale we are breathing out tiny droplets of moisture from deep within. And especially when we sleep, there are several uninterrupted hours to eliminate through the breath. And the modern body is especially loaded with toxins that need to be eliminated. Is it any wonder we wake with 'morning breath'?

~ EXERCISE ~

Oil Pulling

TIME: 5- 20 mins

FREQUENCY: Daily

TOOLS: Sesame, coconut or other cold-pressed oil

METHOD: First thing upon waking, take a mouthful or table spoon of oil. Use sesame oil for the traditional Ayurvedic, negative energy absorbing effect, coconut oil for an antibacterial effect. Really any virgin oil will do. Hold in your mouth with lips closed for at least five minutes. The longer the better. If you work your way up to twenty minutes you will get the most benefit. Gently swill around, pull through teeth and generally allow it to get into every nook and cranny. Spit in the toilet, rubbish bin or garden. It will have increased in volume and become milky white. What you spit out is the toxin laden waste, so be careful not to swallow any. Rinse with warm water and begin your day. This enforced silent time is an ideal opportunity to contemplate, you can combine with palming, earthing or sunning.

Ticks all the boxes!

▶ Simple ✓   ▶ Cheap ✓   ▶ Fast ✓   ▶ Effective ✓

BODY

The one vehicle you have for life

CHAPTER 8

❖

What Cats Know

If you pick up (a relaxed) cat, they flop. They are malleable, flexible and pliable. They are also super gymnasts that can go from complete relaxation to thirty foot up a tree in less than a second. Instant and complete power where and when it is needed. Their trick? Have you noticed, that when not sleeping, they are stretching? Licking this. Washing that. Twisting around under and over. Then, total relaxation. For around twenty-three and a half hours a day.

A dog on the other hand is more like a human. If you pick up a dog, they go stiff. Awkward. The legs are all stiff. Like us, their muscles are 'on' most of the time. Not fully relaxed like their feline cousins. Not 'bag of bones' relaxed. And apart from the occasional downward dog, and an awkward attempt to gnaw at a flea that ends with a comical overbalance, you don't see them doing much stretching.

Now don't get your kitty litter in a mess, I am generalising. I am sure there are dogs who have a ballerina like flexibility. That can leap small buildings in a single bound. But generally speaking...

Stretching is more important than exercise. Okay, there I said it! All these gym bunnies loading their abs, locking their quads and blasting their flab are overlooking one very important thing. Being toned, tight and *inflexible* does not feel good. Does not even look that good. And is a recipe for disaster. Spending fifty-nine minutes on the treadmill and one-minute stretching is what I'm talking about. One day that toned, taut and terrific body will go down in a heap.

Muscles need to breathe. We are constantly using and abusing them. Overuse. Repetition. Inactivity. All cause hardening, tightening and inflexibility. When in spasm, oxygen does not circulate. Waste is not removed. It is an injury waiting to happen.

As you stretch, you let go of tension. There is no 'goal' to reach. No record to break. It is a letting go. An immersion into your inner self. A curious, mental touch-point with every part of your body. How am I *here* today? What does it feel like *now*? Is this side the same as the other? If I breathe and let go how does that feel?

It feels awesome. There is nothing like the feel of a truly stretched body. Forget ten years younger, you will soon feel twenty years younger! And you will move with grace and ease. Lithe and agile like a gazelle. Not lumpy and rigid like a hippopotamus.

~ EXERCISE ~

Stretch

Start stretching. Properly. Daily. You will feel younger. You will move younger. You will look younger. Guaranteed.

TIME: 10 mins

FREQUENCY: Daily

TOOLS: None really necessary but you might like to use a yoga mat or blocks to help with some stretches.

METHOD: Go for all the major muscles you use. Salute to the sun is a lovely sequence to start with. First one salute sequence very slow, holding each position for twenty to thirty seconds. Then three salute sequences fast.

The rules:

- Hold each pose for sixty to ninety seconds. (Yes -*ninety!*).
- No pain. If it ever hurts – stop!
- Breathe. If you hold your breath you aren't allowing the stretch to happen.
- Let go. Of everything. Competition. Achievement. Anger.
- Be curious. You won't get bored if you start to notice... Imbalances. Tighter areas, looser areas. Left side/right side differences. Differences from the last time you

stretched. Feelings. No judgement here, just noticing.It's all part of the process.

Ticks all the boxes!

▶ Simple ✓   ▶ Cheap ✓   ▶ Fast ✓   ▶ Effective ✓

CHAPTER 9

In Defence of the Womb

You know those ads for period pain relief? The one where the balled up, bleeding woman is miraculously bouncing on a tennis court, jogging and skydiving? *Don't do it.* Not the medication. The bouncing. Our grandmothers, traditional cultures, the wise women of old knew a thing or two about their wombs. Menstruating women used to 'remove themselves'. Of course, the feminist in us says: "I can do anything you can do better. And harder. And faster. And whether I'm bleeding or not. And of course you *can*. But come down off your equal opportunity horse for a moment and think about what is going on inside your amazing (and decidedly *un*-male) body.

We women are lucky. Once a month we have an internal system that allows us to get rid of a months' worth of accumulated toxins. We have a brilliant system whereby we can remove, through our blood, any accumulated toxins. We also have our bladders and bowels. We sweat and shed skin. But as women we get a bonus. We have a uterus. What an awesome organ.

And I don't mean awesome in the "I'll have fries with that!" sense. I mean AWEsome. I mean be in awe. What an organ!

First of all, for most of the month it is sitting quietly, the size of a walnut, minding its own business. It lies, suspended by guy-ropes (aka ligaments), deep within your belly. All of a sudden, it's 'that time of the month' and things begin to change. Over the course of a few days it goes from walnut to watermelon (warning: comparisons may vary from reality).

Now remember those guy-ropes? Well they are now suspending an organ that has grown two to three times its weight. These ligaments are all that keep it from dropping right out through your vagina. (BTW, that's called prolapse. Nursing homes are full of former "I can do anything you can do" feminists, whose guy ropes having given up the ghost. Whose uteruses are now permanently descending out of their vaginas.

I know that's kinda gross. But prolapse surgery is a booming trade with an aging, over fifty percent female population. That and radical hysterectomy, where they just whip the offending organ right out. Snip, snip, thank you very much.

Think about it, next time you grab your gym gear while you're bleeding. I know you *can* do it. But maybe those backward cultures with their strange traditions were on to something. I tell you one thing, most had functioning, intact uteruses right up until death. So okay, there is probably no need to isolate yourself in a grass hut on the outskirts of the village. But perhaps the modern equivalent? Cancel kickboxing. Reschedule your run. Be *gentle* with yourself. Listen to your body. Just turn it down a notch.

Some find their periods such an inconvenience, or so painful, they take medication to stop them coming at all. I think this is a mistake. Would you take something that stopped you doing a poo? Forever? What state do you think your body would be in? I know the mechanics of menstruating are a little different. But do you really think you can mess with the natural system and not have consequences? If you suppress menstruation to avoid pregnancy or the inconvenience look for another solution. And if you suffer from debilitating periods, just know suppression is a Band-Aid, not an answer. Ask the question what is so out of balance in your body that your periods are so crushingly painful?

There are many alternative therapies out there to help you find a solution. Herbal medicine, Mayan abdominal massage, hypnosis. Even dropping the resentment you may feel for your body. When you resent, you are discontent. The pain may not be optional, but the negativity in your mind is. Be curious instead. "What did I do *this* month?" "How can I do it differently?"

~ EXERCISE ~

Menstrual Introspection

TIME: Half an hour

FREQUENCY: Monthly

TOOLS: Pen and paper to record feeling.

METHOD: If your periods are no trouble, show your body respect by reducing vigorous activities. Use the time for introspection instead. How can you nurture, respect and connect with your uterus? Your femininity? This is a perfect time for creativity. And for letting go. What else, along with all this blood, can you let go of? What other toxic things in your life can you shed? Thoughts, feelings, relationships?

If you suffer at this time, become a detective. What is your body trying to tell you? Look at all aspects of your life: diet, exercise, emotions. In general, drink lots of water to replace all that liquid that your body is losing.

If you are approaching, or already in, menopause, embracing this milestone, rather than fearing it, will completely change your experience. Many women living in traditional cultures do not report any of the typical menopausal symptoms. The sort of things our western, youth-worshiping culture expects and takes for granted. But what if these symptoms were more to do with the resistance to sacred time in a woman's life? The fear of becoming 'old' and worthless?

► Simple ✓   ► Cheap ✓   ► Effective ✓

CHAPTER 10

———◆———

What Plants Eat

You think you need to protect your skin with sunscreen? I mean that is what they tell us, right? But think about it. For the entire history of humans, the sun has been our friend. We never had to hide from it before. Undiluted sunlight is necessary for true health. In fact, the lack of sunlight causes chronic, low-grade problems that doctors and sunscreen companies do not link with our current sun phobia.

And forget fake tan. I'm sure in a decade we will be seeing some strange illnesses that won't be connected to that toxic stuff. The same goes for sunscreen. Avoid at all costs. What is that toxic muck you are lathering all over your own and your *child's* body? What is in it? Is it safe? Would you spread it on a piece of toast and eat it? Your body would soon tell you it was poisonous. And that gets absorbed into your bloodstream through your skin. So don't be ignorant. Or naïve (but they *said* it was safe!).

Of course, there is nothing attractive about sun damaged skin. The catcher's mitt hide of a frequent tanner is not a pretty thing. Embrace your natural skin tone. And respect it. Then there is no need to tan just because it is the fashion. And it is just a fashion. Instead of following the fashion, lead it. If we all decided that our natural skin tone, be it ivory or dark, is in fashion, then *we're* in charge. Not them.

Our bodies need full spectrum, unfiltered, natural sunlight. Not through glass. Not through clothes. Not through sunscreen. As do our eyes (see chapter six for info on sun-gazing for eye health). The sunglass myth we have *all* bought into, is behind many vision problems.

I live in one of the hottest and sunniest countries in the world. There is a lot of sun in Australia. Summer. Winter. All the time. I used to be addicted to sunglasses. I couldn't leave the house without them. I would turn the car around if I realised I had forgotten them. I felt I couldn't function without them.

When I found out that my sunglass habit was impacting on my health I had to do a sunglass detox. I went cold turkey and for a few days felt I was being blinded. But funny thing is after that, it was fine. I don't squint. The sunlight does not bother me.

When full spectrum sunlight enters our bodies through the eyes it is absorbed by the pituitary gland, the master gland that governs all hormonal activity in the body. The pituitary governs moods. It governs the immune system. And full spectrum sunlight has nutrients that our pituitary needs. Hypothyroidisms anyone? Depression? Autoimmune diseases? These are all a result of a mal-functioning pituitary gland.

We are living such disconnected lives and some may laugh and ask for proof. But you can only get 'proof' if someone is set to make a heap of money from it. And no-one is making any money from sunlight. In fact, there are vested interests who will make money from your fear of it. Cancer councils around the world are built on money made from selling deadly treatments. Treatments that kill hundreds of thousands of people every year. That rarely cure. Treatments that torture and make the last months of a life unendurable.

But I digress...

Obviously, be sensible. If you are going to the beach on a stinker of a day and you will be in the sun all day, cover up. Wear a wide brimmed hat. If you are on a reflective surface, like water or snow, you may need to use sunscreen and sunglasses. Covering up, burka style, is my solution.

I am not an authority. Just someone who acts from my own logical conclusions and common sense. If you don't have that, please don't look to me for it! Draw your own conclusions.

~ EXERCISE ~

Sunning

TIME: 3-10 mins around the middle of the day

FREQUENCY: Daily

TOOLS: Sunny (private) spot

METHOD: Find an area that you can get exposure to natural sunlight and wearing as few clothes as possible lie down and bask. Cover the face as that skin is more delicate. The best time is in the middle of the day, around 11am-1pm, when the full spectrum of sunlight is available. With my pale skin I spend around ten minutes on my front and back. Someone with darker skin will need a little longer. You're a big girl. I leave it up to you. The signal that you have had enough is when you feel the tiniest tingle. Or just before that. You shouldn't even color up and certainly NEVER the burn. And ideally don't shower for quite a while after sunning. It takes several hours for vitamin D to be fully absorbed through the skin, so don't go washing it off!

Ticks all the boxes!

▶ Simple ✓   ▶ Cheap ✓   ▶ Fast ✓   ▶ Effective ✓

CHAPTER II

Do Shoes Make You Old?

When was the last time that your bare feet touched the surface of the earth? On holiday we do it instinctively. We seek nature. We plunge into it. We lay upon it. We become relaxed, recharged, rejuvenated. What if how fabulous you felt after your trip to Fiji was all to do with having your feet on the sand?

In our modern world it is easy to become disconnected from our bodies. We all live in our heads. From a young age children are encouraged to disconnect from their bodies. Sport is so filled with rules and strategies that a physical activity becomes more of a cerebral one.

Stress. Anxiety. Overwhelm. Headaches. Heart palpitations. All the nervous disorders. And most of the mental ones can in part be attributed to this disconnect. So how, in a modern world, do you connect?

The human body is made up mainly of water and minerals, both of which are excellent conductors of electricity. Over the day we build up a charge from our electro-magnetised surrounds. Wi-Fi. Mobile phones. T.V.s. Microwaves. Synthetic materials. Cars, train and especially planes. Modern life is full of barriers between us and the earth's surface. Shoes. Carpet. Concrete. High rise living. All are unnatural exposure to electro-magnetic fields, disconnection and increase the build-up of this static energy in our bodies.

The good news is the entire surface of the earth is a giant electromagnetic sink. Connecting with this drains the charge that builds up as we buzz through our disconnected day.

~ EXERCISE ~

Earthing

TIME: 5 -10 mins

FREQUENCY: Daily

TOOLS: Bare earth, grass or sand

METHOD: Find a patch of grass or sand that is connected to the earth (a child's sand pit with a plastic lining is *not* connected to the earth). Place your bare feet on it. Relax. Reconnect. Perfect activities to do while Earthing are: Palming, Oil Pulling or Natural Vison Exercises.

Ticks all the boxes!

▶ Simple ✓   ▶ Cheap ✓   ▶ Fast ✓   ▶ Effective ✓

CHAPTER 12

Twenty-five Thousand Times a Day

You can calm yourself down through breath. You can hype yourself up. Fear will change how you breathe, as will pleasure, tiredness and illness. You can control pain with your breath. You can generate emotion. You can convey feelings. After just a few minutes without oxygen the brain will cease to function. Vital does not even begin to describe it. Yet we take it for granted. Abuse and misunderstand it.

How you breathe is a litmus test of how you are living your life in that moment. Are you holding on? Not fully participating? Are you giving and giving and not taking enough? We inhale poorly. We hold. We exhale too much and too often.

Oxygen is needed to repair our cells. With every breath our cells are regenerating, replicating. Eliminating and assimilating. Our breath is the vehicle to transport both energy into the cell and waste out of the cell. We breathe between twenty and thirty thousand times a day. So that is twenty thousand opportunities to get it right.

A well oxygenated body is vibrant. Skin is refreshed. Eyes are bright. Muscles are toned. Each breath is both entirely effortless and ultimately effective. But when stressed, inhalation is restricted. Our lungs only expand to a fraction of their capacity. And yes, we can get by on that. But there is a world of difference between surviving and thriving. Stress robs us of our ability to breathe effectively. Waste accumulates. Nutrients are not circulated efficiently. To the brain, the muscles, and the organs. This is why stress is such an insidious disease. It impacts upon such a simple yet vital act, which underpins your entire health.

The tiny muscles between your ribs (intercostal muscles) need to separate to allow you to take a full breath. When these muscles are tight their ability to stretch apart is limited. When they become soft and flexible it is easy to breathe in all that life has to offer you. And like any stretching, it is just a matter of practising.

~ EXERCISE ~

Deep Breathing

TIME: 3 minutes

FREQUENCY: Daily

TOOLS: A quiet place to lie down

METHOD: Lie on your back with your hands placed over your lowest ribs, middle fingers just touching. The goal is to expand the ribs using a gentle, natural breath to create a gap between the tips of your middle fingers. The larger the gap the more you are stretching those ribs. The more space you are creating for your lungs. The breath should not be forced, but gentle, natural and sustainable. It will be slower than normal and slightly elongated.

At first you will barely notice any movement. But over time the intercostal muscles will soften and become more flexible. It will become second nature to breathe fully.

Ticks all the boxes!

▶ Simple ✓   ▶ Cheap ✓   ▶ Fast ✓   ▶ Effective ✓

⬤━━━━⬤━━━━⬤

CHAPTER 13

Green is the New Black

I first heard about green smoothies from Victoria Boutenko in 2003. I will admit I thought it sounded a bit weird. But I listened because I liked a lot of what she shared. At the end of the seminar they handed around a taster of this green drink. It looked scary. But it tasted AMAZING! I was hooked from that moment. That was thirteen years ago. So, why are they all the rage now? What is it about green smoothies that makes them the answer to everything?

Well, to begin with they are GREEN. We don't have much that is green in the Standard Western Diet (SAD). Token. Over cooked. Tasteless. Pretty much useless. Countless studies have shown that cultures with large amounts of greens in their diet experience lower rates of cancer, heart disease and diabetes. Those three diseases that are the curse of the modern world.

So, what is it about greens that is so special?

If you make a green smoothie correctly it is like having a blood transfusion of nutrients. Pure, immediately available and perfectly assimilated.

Green leafy plants are unique in their almost magical ability to take sunlight and transform it into something edible. Eating greens is the closest you can get to eating the pure energy of the sun. Fruits, tubers and stalks are also made from that energy, but it is second-hand. And by the time it gets to the animals you eat, it is third-hand.

Green smoothies are also the answer to expensive (often questionable) vitamins supplements. If you do take supplements, pause for a moment to wonder: what is in them? Have you ever been to a supplement making factory? Just how 'natural' is it? Where do they get it from? How many other unlisted substances are added? Do we need a billion-dollar industry to turn nature into a pill and serve it to us in a plastic container with a price tag?

Green smoothies are incredibly nutrient dense. B vitamins, magnesium. The best source of calcium on the planet (dairy does not even come close - did you know that to absorb calcium you need to consume the correct ratio of magnesium at the same time? So if you have dairy with no magnesium you won't even absorb the calcium. Unlike dairy, guess what green leafy vegies have? You guessed it, the exact ratio of magnesium to calcium for perfect absorption!)

That's not all. Chlorophyll is the ultimate detoxer. In our modern life we are exposed to multiple toxins. It is nearly impossible to avoid. Chemicals in our food. In our water. In our soaps and perfumes. In our air. You can minimise your exposure, but it's pretty much impossible to avoid it completely. The chlorophyll in dark green leafy vegies acts as a natural mopping-up agent. It absorbs and allows us to eliminate those toxins that we are exposed to.

Then there is the fibre. Another thing we have far too little of in our diets. The best fibre comes from your food, not a container. Greens are a beautiful source of gentle fibre that will bulk up your stool, but not bind you up. It will also help to slow down the absorption of sugar by the pancreas.

And then there is sugar cravings and weight loss in general. Much of the time, cravings come from a 'lack' in our diet. Whatever it is, that craving is telling us something is missing. Sugar cravings become a thing of the past, as your body is sated through the nutrient dense cocktail you are offering it. Extra grazing. Unnecessary. Second helpings? Chocolate? They become choices not compulsions.

Your skin starts to take on a radiant glow as a result. Collagen is replenished with the quality, highly available nutrients. Your eyes become clearer with whiter whites. Broken capillaries heal as your body is provided with the natural building blocks for repair.

So why can't we just EAT a ton of greens? Well, unless you want to sit there all day chewing like a cow, you won't be able to break down the tough cell walls of the leaves so as to release all the nutrients.

And having them raw means that you get the live enzymes and the entire nutritional profile, which any heating would compromise.

So, let's see... How *could* we consume large amounts of raw, broken-down, dark-green leafy vegies? Hmmmm... The green smoothie is the perfect solution!

There are a few rules however.

First: Use only LEAFY greens. That means no stalks (like celery), not even the stalks of your kale or chard.

Second: no vegetables like broccoli, cucumber or zucchini. So the perfect green smoothie is made with only the *leafy* part of greens.

Stalks and other vegies are *starchy*. They require clashing digestive enzymes to break them down. This clash of enzymes means your digestive system will be working overtime. You may even have mild reactions such as gas or bloating. However, fruit combines *perfectly* with green leafy vegetables.

The fruit is there to make the smoothies delicious as well as nutritious. And I do mean *delicious*. Not just tolerable. I don't believe in fads. To get the full benefit, it has to be an addition to your diet that is sustainable. If you are not salivating at the thought of drinking your daily green smoothie, then you won't get the full benefit. You may do it for a day or two. Or a week. But forever? Doubtful.

So there it is. Digestion: happy. Bowels: active. Pancreas: happy. Immune system: powered. Energy levels: high. Skin: radiant.

Bones: strengthened. Muscles: relaxed. Detoxification: happening. Cravings: Gone. Are you starting to see why green smoothies are the answer to all ailments?

~ EXERCISE ~

Green Smoothie

TIME: 5 – 10 mins

FREQUENCY: Daily

TOOLS: Dark green leafy vegies, fruit and a good quality blender

METHOD: Make your smoothie daily and *chew* rather drink for best absorption! Smoothies will last for up to 3 days in the fridge, but best consumed on the day. Start with a twenty/eighty combo (fruit being the main part). Work your way to an eighty/twenty combo over time.

Ticks all the boxes!

▶ Simple ✓   ▶ Cheap ✓   ▶ Fast ✓   ▶ Effective ✓

CHAPTER 14

Take with a Pinch of Salt

We are going to get down and dirty now and address the topic of body odour. The smell your body gives off is a message to you. And if it is a nasty message, then it's something you have to listen to.

It is a confronting thing to realise you are a bit 'on the nose'. It is even worse if you are not even aware of it. But spraying, perfuming or suppressing is not the way. First thing is to try to understand *why*. What is out of balance? Is it your diet? Emotions? What about sleep patterns, are they off? Are stress levels through the roof?

Then take action. You need to look at those issues and see where you can make adjustments. Take control, rather than being at the mercy. Change your diet. Monitor your stress levels and put things into place to change lifestyle to support yourself. Because if you do not listen to your body now, eventually it will *force* you to listen. Where do you think years, decades, of ignoring the small, harmless messages (like smell) will get you?

When using any deodorant under your arms, choose carefully. It is a highly absorptive area. And it is in close proximity to the lymph glands. And your breast. Do you know what waxed or shaved skin looks like under the microscope? Tiny lesions. Now think about this:

Lesions → poison (antiperspirant) → lymph nodes → breast tissue

What does that add up to? I'm no federally-funded cancer council, but I'd hazard a guess it couldn't be good. So be smart and opt out of antiperspirant use before the *official* announcement comes about the dangers come out.

But no one wants to be smelly, so what to do? Odour is caused by bacteria that loves moist, dark areas (armpits anyone?). A simple, effective answer is to make the environment bacteria-*un*friendly. And the way to do that is with salt. Bacteria and salt do not like each other. That's why salt is used to preserve meat. A salt-brine deodorant will keep your armpits, and any other area you wish to apply it to, smelling sweet. And it is one hundred percent safe. You can even drink it if you want.

~ EXERCISE ~

Salt Brine Deodorant

TIME: Once brine is made, just a few seconds

FREQUENCY: 2 x daily

TOOLS: Unrefined salt of choice, purified water. Glass spray bottle.

METHOD: To make the brine, dissolve around a quarter of a cup of unprocessed natural salt in a litre of warm (not hot) water. The stronger the better. Spray liberally under arms after your shower. Use on its own or add a few drops of your favourite essential oils for scent. You may need to kill bacteria you already have with a few drops of diluted Teatree oil. After that you should be able to keep the sour odour at bay simply by applying a salty brine solution on clean armpits twice a day.

Ticks all the boxes!

▶ Simple ✓   ▶ Cheap ✓   ▶ Fast ✓   ▶ Effective ✓

CHAPTER 15

(Almost) Better than Sex

King Henry had one. So did the Queen of the Nile. You can become one yourself. But why would anyone want to be a poooligist? Not of anyone else's poo. But of your own. What better way to know *exactly* what is going on inside you than to understand the nature of what is coming out of you?

Forget expensive and invasive MRIs, x-rays or blood tests. Just look at your poo. That's right. I said *look* at it? Be curious. Because there is a wealth of information there if you are willing to look. So don't be scared; don't be precious. Be curious. We all do it. Your bowel is your body's main method of elimination. If you want to know how effective your system is; start looking.

So what *is* the Perfect Poo? You need to answer that for yourself. I am my own poooligist. You need to become yours. I know what is perfect for me. You need to find out what is perfect for you. Don't hand your power over to the experts. It's *your* poo. Become your own expert. Here are some things to look for.

- **Frequency**. How often is good for you? And how often is perfect? Once a day. Two times? How often is too often? What is too infrequent? And what changes the frequency? Stress? Anxiety? Diet? For me it is one 'proper' poo a day.

- **Duration**. How long does it take to evacuate? Is it an explosive rush? Or are you taking in a newspaper (or your phone) and settling in for a good long browse? Perfect for me is a five seconds. I'm happy if it takes me less time to poo than to wee.

- **The wipe.** Is it messy? Is it clean? Do you need to use half a role of loo paper? For me, perfect is a Teflon poo. Do I need to explain?

- **Consistency**. You may have seen the poo chart. There is a whole 'science in' itself. Corn-on-the-cob or porridge? Bunch of grapes or sausage? Floats or sinks? I'm not here to tell you what is *right* or *wrong* because when you start noticing I am sure you can work it out. The key is to start noticing patterns and then you can interpret.

- **Effort**. Straining? Giving birth? Pain? The less effort the better, I'd say.

- **Smell**. It is poo, it's going to smell. But is it weird? Chemical? Nasty or 'normal'? Is it foul to the point of passing out? Notice, because this will change and is a direct message about what is going on inside.

- **Completion**. How do you feel after? Is there a sense of completion? Or do you still feel like there is unfinished business?

As the Royal poooligist you needed a strong constitution. And not just because of all that smelling. Imagine informing your king, who had a head-lopping fetish that his crap stank.

~ EXERCISE ~

The Perfect Poo

TIME: Moments is all it takes

FREQUENCY: Each time you go!

TOOLS: Eyes and ears. And nose.

METHOD: So now you have the criteria. Become your own poooligist and see what your body is telling you. Start to notice. Be curious. Get to know your body. Do you need to adjust your diet? Is stress taking a toll on your internals? How can you help?

Ticks all the boxes!

▶ Simple ✓   ▶ Cheap ✓   ▶ Fast ✓   ▶ Effective ✓

CHAPTER 16

Where We All Came From

'Vagina' is not a term bandied about in polite company. We are so disconnected from 'down there' we can't even say its name. Being disconnected from a major organ, especially the one that defines your womanhood, is crazy. But so many are. A friend of mine had such painful periods. Every month was days of hell. Cramps. Blood clots. Pain. She would take to her bed with hot water bottles and painkillers. She *hated* her womb and all it stood for. When something causes you that much pain it's natural to disconnect from it. It is not a fun place to be. Energetically. Emotionally. But if you go down that path what other issues are you creating? Sex. Conception. Pregnancy. Labour. Hating a part of your body that is intrinsically involved in such major events is a recipe for disaster. Challenges in conception. Issues with sex. Difficult pregnancies. The answer may be as simple as restabilising a relationship with your womb.

If you want to reclaim and reconnect then you will love the vaginal steam. Also known as the *yoni bath*, this ancient Mayan method has been used for centuries to address disorders, to tone and to heal. From menstrual irregularities to menopausal symptoms. From infertility or to fibroids. Instead of ignoring, supressing or even removing our wombs, this technique brings back the sacredness.

And it's simple: steeped herbs are placed in hot water, you sit above and the medicinal vapours are absorbed through your vaginal tissues.

~ EXERCISE ~

Vaginal Steam (AKA Under Carriage Steam Clean)

TIME: 10 – 20 mins

FREQUENCY: As needed, but monthly around a week prior to menstruation.

TOOLS: Heat proof bowl, herbs, blanket.

METHOD: Boil a handful of your chosen fresh or dried herbs for ten minutes. Allow them steep for another five minutes. Place the liquid in a heat proof bowl that you have reserved for just this purpose. It must be large enough to be wedged into the toilet without slipping down. Toilet must be clean and free from any cleaning chemical residue. It's a delicate area, so BE CAREFUL! You may need to add some cold water if the steam is too scalding. Remove underpants sit on the toilet seat with the hot bowl under you. Wrap up well, use a blanket to keep the warmth in and draughts out.

Relax for ten to twenty minutes. Allow the vapors to rise and absorb. It is the most incredible feeling. Of course do not do if you have any lesions or open wounds. And never use essential oils.

The herbs you can use are many and varied. I suggest you do your own research.

A few that are easy to get and have multiple benefits are-

- **Rosemary** - cleanse, circulation
- **Lavender** - calming
- **Oregano** - brings on menses if scanty or irregular
- **Marigold** - cleanse, wound healing
- **Basil** - painful periods, scar tissue (i.e. episiotomy)

Different conditions will require different schedules. Consult with your natural health care provider for a personalised plan.

▶ Simple ✓   ▶ Cheap ✓   ▶ Effective ✓

MIND

Your Thoughts Are Real Forces

CHAPTER 17

Why this Daily Routine Ages You

Ok, here is one to give you back your time. And dignity. Stop consuming 'NEWS'. You know what news stands for? N.E.W.S = Negative Energy Well Spoken. This toxic information is slickly packaged and delivered in such a way that we are made to feel guilty if we *don't* partake. Uninformed. Ignorant. How insulting! The news is cleverly formatted entertainment, designed to make you feel like you are 'participating' in local and world events. As though you are a *responsible* member of society. When in reality you are not. You are simply being bludgeoned over the head with controversial, salacious, violent, sexual, racist or bigoted views. And ads.

The lowest common denominator is catered to. The ignorant. The disenfranchised. The rapists and murderers. This is *their* platform. Why do intelligent, kind, normal people buy into it? This is not *my* world.

No matter what side of an argument you fall on you will either feel vindicated or outraged. And this emotional state is what will help the radio station, TV network or online news source sell more pizza. Or overseas holidays. Or aluminium siding. Don't be fooled, it is just a devious attempt to sell advertising space. Or prop up a network with a sheen of respectability. The saying "If it bleeds, it leads" is real.

And how does it make you feel? Self-righteous? Depressed? Angry? Guilty? Slightly nauseated? Don't you have enough to worry about? This is a toxin in your mind. Do you want network managers deciding what thoughts you think? Has it ever (be honest), *ever* moved you to go out and make a difference?

So it is time to detox.

You can do it. And none of this weaning yourself off. Go cold turkey and free up your mind with one fell swoop. If you wish to be informed about an issue, do your own research. Find differing views and create your own opinion. Don't become a patsy to this savvy marketing machine.

At Easter, a friend of mine was all of a fluster. Apparently so as not to offend any Muslims, they were ban hot cross buns!

Now Marge is a mild-mannered, middle-class matron in her eighties. She goes to church every Sunday. She knits knick-knacks to raise money for children in Africa. But how could a good woman like her *not* have a reaction to such inflammatory announcement? Her radio station had her up in arms and ready to run an ethnic group out of town. She had been manipulated (with a lie) into feeling the way the radio station wanted her to feel. They had helped her develop a strong dislike for a group of people she had had nothing to do with in her middle-class, white-bread life.

So here it is. *They* have an agenda. They *want* you to feel a certain way. Why? Because emotion is addictive. And encourages purchasing. And because we, the listener, actually *like* that feeling of outrage. For example, I am *enjoying* the feeling of outrage *I* have for the shock jocks and the news in general. It makes me feel superior. It makes me feel justified. And if life is a bit boring, it is a safe place to vent and rage. Then it's back to the knitting.

Everything that you allow to enter your mind leaves a stain. Like putting a drop of dye into a clear pool, if you do it over and over and over, the clear water will start to take on the color. Do you want the powers that be at radio station 'xyz' deciding what is in *your* mind? Making their agenda yours? This stuff is dangerous in the wrong hands. We are not all as mild mannered as Marge, and some harmless huffing and puffing may not be the only result.

In the movie 'Bowling for Columbine' Michael Moore put forward the theory that the mass shootings that the USA is well known for, were caused by the media. He made a very good argument for it, and I do not know if it is true or not, but think on this. If several times a day you hear about atrocities being committed in the Middle East, a Muslim doing a dastardly deed, a suspicious sighting of a man of Middle Eastern appearance, another Middle Eastern atrocity, and a story about a local council that wants a mosque to be built. Where is your mind by the end of the day? Now times that by fifty-two days. How are you feeling about the Middle Eastern community? Have you any bias? Is it based on reality, or is it coloured by what the networks want you to think?

You may think you are being 'well informed' by listening or watching the news, but you have simply been indoctrinated into their way of thinking. Influenced. Swayed. If you think you don't get affected by it, try this exercise; when driving try *not* to read any advertisements. NONE. Bus, billboard or bakery sign. It takes a huge amount of concentration. So who has control of what is going into your mind? Can you be surrounded, immersed and yet remain unpolluted? Because I very much doubt it. If you can - congrats, it takes control to not be stained by your surroundings.

There are atrocities being committed every day everywhere. I am sure we could find atrocities being committed by all religions and creeds. It is sad. Does hearing about it over and over and over and over mean that you will go out there and make a difference?

So, you do have a choice. You don't *have* to listen. You can turn it off.

~ EXERCISE ~

News Embargo

TIME: This one gives you *back* time!

FREQUENCY: Daily

TOOLS: Remote control, self-discipline

METHOD: TURN IT OFF. Try a week with NO NEWS. How does that feel? If you are fearful that the world might explode and you won't hear about it, believe me, you will have plenty of well-meaning friends to fill you in. They love it when *they* get to be the one breaking the breaking news!

When you rarely see or hear the news delivered in an urgent monotone by a suit-wearing talking head, it is much easier to see it for what it is: *info-tainment*. So if you can't go cold turkey and immediately stop this time-wasting, mind numbing, politically biased habit – then try weaning yourself off. First cut down to only watching, listening or reading the 'news' once a day. Then once a week. Pretty soon you will see it for what it is, a biased account of events told in a way to generate a reaction and get you incensed.

That does not mean that you need to be uninformed. But be proactive and inform *yourself*. Read or watch in-depth investigative journalism pieces, which still have their own bias, but will give you much more of the whole story than the puerile tat served up nightly at six pm.

Ticks all the boxes!

► Simple ✓   ► Cheap ✓   ► Fast ✓   ► Effective ✓

CHAPTER 18

The Power of Dark

I spent an interesting evening with my two raucous nephews on World Energy Day a few years ago. We turned off all electrical appliances at seven pm, and lit a few candles. The result was amazing. The boys assumed a hushed tone. Dinner was decidedly low key, just gentle conversation. They had no desire to race about in their usual pre-bed fashion. They cuddled up for bed time stories and slid into effortless sleep.

You may think 'the perfect sleep' is a dream. Or that you need sleeping pills to achieve it. You know, a sleep where you lay down, fall asleep within thirty seconds then awake six or seven hours later having barely moved a muscle, refreshed and raring to go? Is it only a dream?

There is nothing so wonderful as to wake feeling completely refreshed. To wake *before* the alarm. To be full of energy, ready to face the day. If you know *how* to sleep its half the battle won.

One trick is sleeping in total darkness. It involves a trip to a curtain store for blackout curtains and trip to a tip to throw away your digital clock. Any light that enters will disrupt the delicate circadian rhythms. And they are so often disrupted in our modern, unnatural lives that they need all the help they can get. Street light, moonlight or starlight sneaking through the curtain gaps may be romantic but they disrupt a completely restful sleep that total darkness allows.

So, curtains closed, now the test. Can you see your hand in front of your face? Yes? Then it's too light. It needs to be pitch dark. And try to avoid night time toilet trips by reducing your liquid intake before bed. If you do have to go, do not turn on any lights. When any light enters your eyes it plays havoc with your internal sleep cycles. Your body goes into full alert, then when you get back into bed, it just confuses everything. You are now training your body to ignore the message of seeing light. Which is not a good habit if you want to wake refreshed.

So tinkle in the dark, go on, I dare you! It is much easier than you think. Unless you have set up an obstacle course between your bed and the toilet I am sure you can manage. And if you really don't trust yourself then have the lowest wattage, smallest size night light and when in the loo, don't be tempted to turn on the overhead lights either.

The best sleep comes from having a caffeine free body. I don't mean no coffee after 5pm. I mean none, ever. I'm not about to start on with the whole no caffeine debate. I'm just saying. Have you (ever) gone a day, two days, a week without caffeine? (Cola, coffee, tea, green tea, chocolate etc.) Ever? Think about it.

Try going for three weeks with no sugar or caffeine. (Did you see that? I slipped that other addictive substance in there!). The sleep you will experience will be sublime. With no stimulants racing about your body (maybe for the first time ever) you can really switch off. One hundred percent off. And the truly amazing thing is that most people will never get to experience - when you sleep so well, you wake so refreshed that you don't *need* that coffee to kick start you. You are naturally started. Fresh and ready to go. It is a beautiful thing to experience.

Another thing that helps is to sleep a little cooler than you think you need to. Not too much, just a little. Take off that extra blanket. If you are worried about being too cool, wear socks.

If you habitually find you can't get off to sleep this is certainly affecting your ability to wake refreshed. It happens occasionally to all of us, especially if there has been a stressful event that plays on your mind. But if it is just the way you are every night, then you need to look at what you are doing in the lead up to bedtime.

If you are a parent, you will know that stimulation before bedtime is not good. Warm baths, a soothing bedtime story are the order of the day. Imagine if there was rough and tumble, loud music and sugary food. Would you expect tears when you plopped your child into bed after that? Resistance? Toys thrown about the room?

The adult equivalent is that racing mind, obsessing, lit up like a Christmas tree when all you want is to float away. So treat yourself like a baby. No stimulation for several hours before bed. Oh and no alcohol, that is a stimulant too. Boring isn't it. Hey, I didn't call this chapter sleep dark and have fun.

What constitutes stimulation? TV obviously, there is nothing like hearing the state of the world to give you nightmares. And most movies are designed to stir emotions; happiness, joy, sadness, depression. Even the light of the TV, your phone or iPad will stimulate.

~ EXERCISE ~

Sleep Dark

TIME: This one gives you *back* time!

FREQUENCY: Every night

TOOLS: Blackout curtains

METHOD: as well as installing blackout curtains and making sure your room is in total darkness, create an evening routine. What can you do to calm rather than stimulate?

- Make your bedroom a TV and phone free zone
- No caffeine
- No liquids few hours before bed
- Gentle stretching.
- Warm shower or bath
- Soft music
- Muted lighting
- No screens
- Reading (nothing too stimulating)
- Meditation
- Affirmations
- Journaling
- Listen to a relaxation track
- Breathing exercises

Ticks all the boxes!

▶ Simple ✓   ▶ Cheap ✓   ▶ Fast ✓   ▶ Effective ✓

CHAPTER 19

Words Change Everything

Dr. Masaru Emoto demonstrated an interesting phenomenon of how energy effects matter with water. Frozen water is looked at under the microscope and is made up of millions of tiny crystals. The microscopic crystals are affected by emotion. By energy. By words. Some words create broken, misshapen crystals within the water. Some create perfect, symmetrical crystals.

This stuff may sound strange, but your thoughts affect your world. How? Because our thoughts have an energy that resonates and that resonance has an effect. You can change the 'energy' of what you put in, or on, your body by blessing it?

What does what you say have to do with what you eat? Have you ever made a meal when angry? Or eaten one when angry? What about when you're happy? Does it change the taste of the food? Would you want to eat angry energy? Hateful, depressed energy? So how do you eat positive energy instead? Simple. A few seconds prior to eating give the thought of gratitude. Of health. Of love.

I know that I want whatever is going into my body to be made of whole, symmetrical structures that resonate with the energy of gratitude, love and peace. Rather than something made of deformed, fractured crystals and resonating with the energy of anger, sadness or stress.

It does take some awareness to wait those few moments before you hoe in. A few moments to think thoughts of gratitude. But if my food changes its molecular structure to something whole and pure, then I'm all for it. I think that our thoughts have more of an effect on the safety of our food than the organic-ness or GMO-ness does.

Where does cancer come from? The pharmaceutical companies and doctors don't have a clue, do they? I mean smoking doesn't help (obviously), but it is not a direct line from smoking to cancer, is it? Every single smoker doesn't get cancer. What if the molecular structure of the food you eat (which is directly affected by the words you say and the thoughts you think) is creating an environment for cancer to thrive in or be repelled from?

That really is food for thought!

~ EXERCISE ~

Food Blessing

TIME: 30 seconds

FREQUENCY: Every time you eat

TOOLS: a short sentence you can recite

METHOD: Take a few moments to express gratitude for your food by 'blessing' it. To whomever. God, if that is your thing. The farmers. Your husband. It does not really matter. The energy of your thoughts is gratitude. Feeling blessed that placing food in your mouth is a daily occurrence. Thoughts of abundance and health.

Find an easy to remember blessing that resonates with you, that you can utter quietly, or not, before eating.

Ticks all the boxes!

▶ Simple ✓   ▶ Cheap ✓   ▶ Fast ✓   ▶ Effective ✓

CHAPTER 20

How to Stack the Deck

What is the deal with everyone's acceptance of killing insects? And fish? I cannot understand why someone thinks it is okay to stomp on the head of a spider. Or commit a cockroach to a slow death of asphyxiation. Or to jab a hook through a fish's mouth and drown it for pleasure. Try this to see if you get where I'm coming from. Replace the word *fish* with *calf*. Or the word *spider* with *squirrel*. *Cockroach* with *puppy*. You would NEVER! And the people who did would be considered insane. They say that psychopaths usually torture animals before they move on to people.

Why is a cockroach's life worth less than a hummingbird? Would you slap your shoe on a hummingbird? Why not? So don't be racist, or should I say *animal-ist*. If you think some insects or fish are more worthy than others, have a chat to their mothers. Or to them. Do you think they want to die at your hands? They feel pain. Maybe because you can't hear their screams or recognise the terror in their eyes, you think they are okay with being killed. Well, shame on you.

So here is the question, how is not killing insects going to make you look younger? Have you ever glimpsed your face in the mirror as you are about to smash the life out of something? No? Well take a look next time. It ain't pretty. You have much the same expression when exterminating an ant as you would if you were pulling a gun on someone. There is hatred. Anger.

Okay, but here is the REAL reason. It is steeped in an ancient belief. The belief is that every energetic action you bring into the world with your mind, your voice or your body creates a wave that resonates and is returned to you. Call it karma. Call it what goes around comes around. Call it 'do unto others'. You get the picture. Well, when you take another being's life, and yes, ants are beings. As are moths. And blowflies. That energy is reflected back to you in the form of shortening *your* lifespan as well as creating illness and bad health.

So if you let (or worse, encourage!) your children to kill, you are shortening their lives and helping them to create the causes for illness and bad health.

I have not killed a mozzie in over twenty years. I have killed ants inadvertently when they get washed down the sink. But I have rescue missions in place to help them if I get to them in time. I do not live in a house that is overrun with cockroaches. Or mice. Or ants. Mossies no longer are interested in me. Whereas they make a bee line for my friends who are swatting them mercilessly. What is with that?

I think that fear and killing energy actually attracts the pests. And I guarantee I have less insects, spiders, cockroaches, flies in my house than the people who go about spraying, stomping and poisoning. It is laughable to think that the one blowfly you just smashed the life out of will mean your house is cleaner, more sanitary. There are a billion, trillion others just outside waiting to come in. And you have created a vacuum. And the energy of killing has now entered your home. Worse it has entered into your body where it is now aging you and your cells.

~ EXERCISE ~

Insect Removal

TIME: Only a minute or two!

FREQUENCY: As needed

TOOLS: Spider catcher, ant catcher etc.

METHOD: So how to deal with the unwanted visitors?

You will need to make several different insect catching devices and have them scattered about the house. For ants a pastry brush and a small plastic container is ideal. Gently brush them into the container and place them outside.

For bigger critters; spiders, cricket cockroaches, a bigger container and a stiff thin piece of board to slide under. Again place them outside. Brooms can also be used to shepherd spiders out of windows.

There are humane traps for rats/mice that catch but do not kill. You then 'relocate' them. Yes, it takes some effort. Possums in the roof can also be relocated. In Australia we have a business called 'possum busters' and they come in and create a one way opening out of your roof so they get out and they cannot get back in. If you want to be super kind you can also get them to put a box up in a nearby tree so they have a new home to relocate to.

Deterrents are better than removal. Tea-tree oil, cinnamon oil, citronella oil, pennyroyal oil. These can be sprinkled or sprayed about where insects like to come. It is usually enough to keep them at bay. And your house will smell glorious.

It is up to you but be aware that if you deprive another of its life there will be consequences. So long as you are happy to own those consequences, go right ahead. It does take too much effort to have a peaceful coexistence with your fellow beings. And respect for other's lives is such a beautiful thing that reflects in your face.

Ticks all the boxes!

► Simple ✓   ► Cheap ✓   ► Fast ✓   ► Effective ✓

CHAPTER 21

Put Your Doctor Out of Business

Most people have the wrong idea about meditation. Let me tell you what it is not. It is *not* having your mind be empty of all thoughts. Not at all. It is *not* being at peace with the world. It is *not* floating off to a land of cherry pies and pink lemonade. It is *not* 'zoning out'. It is *not* inspecting your navel for fluff. These are popular misconceptions.

Meditation is actually an Olympic Games level feat for your mind. It is not for the faint of heart. It is not for the weak of will. You will come face to face with yourself. You will see yourself, perhaps for the first time, for who you *really* are. And for most of us that is confronting. And unexpected. It is taking the mask off to reveal the real you. Warts and all. No bullshit.

Not meditating, we spend most of our lives trying to *avoid* who we really are. We do it with alcohol. With shopping. With TV. With inane social events. With 'busyness'. When you meditate you just sit with yourself. Maybe for the first time you start to know your real self.

Why is that important? Well if you don't know who you are, then how would you know how to grow? What you need? What your strengths are? Your weaknesses? And when you do know the answer to those questions, what do you do with it? How does this information make you look or feel younger?

We are at the mercy of our minds. We see something on TV, on the side of a bus and we have a hair trigger response. We have to look. And that triggers a thought that we have to think it. We worry about this or that. Sleepless nights. Obsessive thoughts. These are things that will age you by the minute. How can you not think that thought? React to that situation? Obsess about that remark? It feels like it is out of your control.

Meditation changes all that. First you meet yourself. It is a strange and interesting encounter. Then you get to know yourself. That is a telling experience. Confronting. Unexpected. Liberating.

Why do we spend most of our life trying very hard not to have this encounter? Why are we so scared of just being with ourselves?

Sit for a while and you may just get the answer.

Why 'waste' this time?

The thing is, in our lives we will all have difficulties. Challenges. Tragedies. You may lose your job. You may lose your husband. Your children may disappoint or shock you.

There will be deaths and departures. There will be heartache and horror.

So if some sadness is a given, why do we spend so much of our life trying to pretend we can somehow escape it? That we are that special snowflake who will not experience tragedy, suffering or unhappiness?

We might think; if I'm rich enough, if my child goes to the right school. If my husband has the right position in the company. If my house is in the right neighbourhood. If I look young enough. If I have the respect, admiration or envy of my friends. If everything is just so! THEN I will be immune to sadness. THEN it will all be okay. THEN I will be finally happy.

Yet, now more than ever, we seek out pharmaceutical, alcoholic or recreational drugs as an inoculation to these feelings. We are busier than ever. We are more disconnected. More distracted. We are afraid of what may be unlocked, if we just *be*. We have devised all manner of ways to escape. On every bus, television, every available surface is a new seduction.

Meditation is the answer. It will give you a case of cold hard reality. After an initial shock you will find it's not all that bad. That just *being* is okay. And when you are able to remain present in the moment, anxiety, depression, dissatisfaction; all melt away.

~ EXERCISE ~

Meditation

TIME: Start with 5 minutes build up to 20.

FREQUENCY: Daily

TOOLS: None necessary but could have quiet/sacred space set up with cushion(s), mat, shawl, timer, candle/incense/ flowers etc.

METHOD: In a safe environment you get to come face to face with yourself. Slowly over time you start to understand how your particular flavor of demons' work. What are your triggers? Your weaknesses? How do you avoid? Deal with pain? And then you simply observe. To the outside world you may be navel gazing and 'wasting time'. Internally you are finding out, probably for the first time, how to deal with discomfort. How to face fear. How to pre-empt pain. How to remain calm in the face of calamity. The beautiful thing is that it is possible. Meditation teaches you how.

Ticks all the boxes!

► Simple ✓   ► Cheap ✓   ► Fast ✓   ► Effective ✓

---·-----·---

CHAPTER 22

Putting it All Together

So can you do all these great techniques, every day? Unlikely! Do I? No! However, one step at a time you can start to incorporate more healthy habits in your life, and start to turn back time. The thing is to make it easier not harder!

The first few hours of your day sets the tone for the whole day. This is precious time. The golden hours when your brain is at its freshest. You have a choice, either time controls you or you control time.

My tip is to create before you consume.

So what is the first thing you do? If it includes checking emails and logging on to social media sites, you are letting others dictate the type of day you will have. If you wake to hear the morning news bulletin, is that really what you want to spend that super brain time on? Stories of doom and gloom, inane talk-back or trashy songs and ads for cars and soft drink?

Don't squander this time on unimportant tasks, procrastinating or rushing about. Set aside at least half an hour *for you*. What you do with that time is up to you, but hitting the snooze button a dozen times may not be the theme you want to create for your day. Unless procrastination and feeling out of control are what you are aiming for.

Decide to give yourself the time. Then work backwards from when you have to leave or start your day. There are many things in this book that could make up your morning routine. I like to include some liquid intake, some sort of exercise and something mental. For example, drench, stretch, meditate.

But there is a ninja hack I have discovered that will actually *create* time! We all know how the morning seems to fly and before you know it you are already running late. So here is the ninja hack; timers!

Set timers on your phone for fifteen or thirty minute intervals. This is how it looks for me: if I'm up at five, first alarm is five fifteen. That first alarm is the most important, because when I get up early I feel like I have all the time in the world. It's easy to day-dream my way through an hour, then, boom, I'm back to having to rush. So in that first fifteen minutes I have to toilet, feed pets, wash, dress and prepare a hot drink. It means I have to really move! The next alarm is at five thirty and so on.

The other trick to creating time in your morning is to start your routine the night before.

First, work out how much sleep your body *naturally* needs. No stimulants. No alarms. And then make sure you give yourself that time. If it is seven hours, then make sure you are in bed seven and a half hours before you want to start your morning. I tend to be a night owl. I resist going to bed early. I faff about and before I know it I am barely in bed before midnight. That makes a five am start a bit painful. So at ten pm I set an alarm for going to bed.

Next, you need to know exactly *what* you will be doing. Have all that you will need for your morning routine ready. Lemon drench; do you have lemons? Stretch: do you have clean yoga pants? Meditation; do you have your cushion and a spot set up? Do you have your body brush? Your journal? Whatever it is you need. Have your routine planned. Have your equipment at hand. Don't waste a second of your precious morning with finding stuff, digging things out or setting yourself up.

If up until now you have allowed you morning routine to be dictated to you by others, isn't it time you took back control? You have a choice. But you have to make it. Because if you are not proactive, the snooze button, the radio stations and the rest of society will easily make the decision for you.

I have devised a twenty-one-day program based on all the techniques. You will find the link to the challenge here: https://app.convertkit.com/landing_pages/46867

~ EXERCISE ~

TIME: 10 mins - 2 hours

FREQUENCY: Daily

TOOLS: Be prepared the night before with whatever equipment you will need.

METHOD: Set up your routine the night before. Have a series of alarms to keep you on track. Set a going to bed alarm, it is amazing how fast time goes early in the morning!

▶ Simple ✓   ▶ Cheap ✓   ▶ Effective ✓

CHAPTER 23

Attitude

I have known twenty-five year olds that could be mistaken for forty year olds. And forty year olds that appeared to be in their twenties. It is not all looks. Having a youthful attitude will shave years off your appearance. So what *is* a youthful attitude? Is it wearing low slung, skin tight jeans and sneering? Is it answering in monosyllabic grunts?

A youthful demeanour is one that is flexible not rigid. That is easy-going not uptight. That is curious not jaded. If you always have to be in control, what do you look like? Do you only want things done your way? Get stressed at the drop of a hat? Think you have seen it all, know it all? If so, no matter your chronological age you will appear at least a decade older than you are.

Changing this attitude is easier said than done. That subconscious need to be in control is a response to deep fear. Fear of losing control or being out of control. It is often so much part of us we cannot imagine anything different. It is a constant gnawing need and it produces stress in our bodies.

And stress is one of the most aging things. Stress is also totally subjective. Happy marriage (but he snores!). Healthy kids (but they don't do things just how *you* want them to). Financially well-off (but there is always the next bright shiny thing). The morning rush. The appointments. The fear of being judged. Having to have things *just so*. Outwardly you may have a perfect life, but inwardly you could be living with a mountain of stress of your own making.

The first thing is to realise it is a choice. And that is not easy to hear. Because, if it really is a choice, then what does that say about you? But this is not a judgemental thing. This is an acceptance thing. Acceptance of yourself and your power to make decisions.

Believe it or not, what goes into your mind is your choice. No one else's. Just yours.

So how to change?

1. **Want to.** That seems a no brainer. But is it? I am amazed how many people get attached to being stressed. It gives them a sense of meaning. Of importance. They actually *like* it. So you need to *want* it.
2. **Notice.** You can't change something until you become aware of it. This is meditation brought into your everyday life. Become the observer of yourself. What triggers that attitude? When does your chest tighten? Your frown start? The judgements (of self and others) jump in?

3. **Replace.** Now you have become aware you have the power to make a choice. Will you or won't you? React. Have your usual response. Or do something different. Let it go. Become curious. Stretch your mind and see what is possible.

4. **Let go.** Of control. This single act is the most vitalizing and youth-giving action. No need for a face-lift when you are prone to softening rather than hardening around an issue. When you are relaxed and okay with what life throws you. And it is sexy too. Few men can resist that balm of relaxation. Try it!

~ EXERCISE ~

Mind Power

TIME: 1 minute

FREQUENCY: Several times a day

TOOLS: Phone alarms and will power

METHOD: Put reminders in your phone several times a day. When the alarm goes off immediately notice what you are thinking and feeling at that very moment. First identify and name the emotion. Next decide if you want to let it go. Then if you do, replace it. With a feeling or thought or visualization or affirmation of your choosing. Soon it will start to become a habit and you won't need the reminders. Your thoughts start to become conscious instead of unconscious.

► Simple ✓   ► Cheap ✓   ► Effective ✓

CHAPTER 24

Special Mentions

Salt

You may think you are being healthy by having a low salt diet, but salt is one of the healthiest, essential elements to life. And excluding it from your diet is counterintuitive. Have a think about it. All the fluids in your body are salty. Your blood. Your sweat. Your tears. Where does that salt come from? We don't manufacture it in house. Animals in the wild will cross deserts, risk their lives to access locations where salt naturally occurs. Farmers provide saltlicks for their stock. So why this madness from the medical system about salt? If our body cannot function without it, then why are we told to avoid it? Why are low (or no!) salt diets the catch-cry of every other doctor?

It comes down to what salt is. There are two types of salt. Real salt, unrefined and containing a multitude of nutrients, and fake salt, highly refined and containing only sodium chloride.

If you eat a diet of processed food, you will be consuming mostly that second type. Fake salt. This is a poison that causes all the angst. Food manufacturers are not silly. They know that salty food is 'more-ish'. And it tastes better. They know that you will compulsively reach for handful after handful of those salted nuts. Whereas you stop after just a few of the unsalted ones. And the same goes for all processed foods. Sauces. Chutneys. Sweet drinks. In fact, sweet drinks like cola or lemonade are so laden with salt it's not even funny. Then they load it up with sugar to make it palatable. The clever thing about the (fake) salt in soda is that it also makes you thirsty. Clever eh?

Refined salt also has another little nasty added. Anti-caking agent. Notice how dry and 'pourable' refined table salt is? (That is the fake one) When you grab the shaker it sprinkles out in an easy fashion. Unrefined salt is quite a different. Often it is damp, it cakes together. It blocks the shaker. That is why they add an anticaking agent. But the anti-caking agent stops salt from being absorbed and causes it build up in the arteries. It is also made of aluminium! I am sure you know how damaging aluminium is. And the iodine they often add to table salt? The anti-caking agent renders it un-absorbable. It is a nightmare.

Lugol's Solution

Iodine is an amazing element. In times gone past it was used to clean wounds and the inside of milk vats. Its residue had surprising health benefits that are more important today than ever. Iodine is one of those under resourced nutrients that protects the thyroid and balances your hormones. And our thyroids need all the help they can get. Anti-bacterial products, hair dyes, fluoride. These, and a million other household products, contain the ion bromide. Bromide attaches to the thyroid gland receptors and cause it to go out of balance. This is a very simplistic explanation of what happens, if you want more in-depth understanding I would encourage you to do your own research. Suffice to say, we do not consume enough iodine through our food. And the crap they add to table salt is a joke as already discussed. Bromides are everywhere and funnily enough, so are thyroid problems. If you consume iodine in the form of the supplement Lugol's solution, you will be knocking out the bromides and giving your thyroid a fighting chance. Available from good health food stores.

Pet Diet

Have you ever seen a cat cook? Have you ever heard of a dog who harvested grain? So why would you think that cooked meat or processed grains are what your pet should eat? This unnatural diet leads to many health issues for our pets. And unfortunately keeps many vets in practice.

There is no such thing as a fussy eater in nature. Nor an overweight animal. These are human conditions brought on by our unnatural diets.

If you want your beloved pet to stay young, longer, think of what they would eat if they were in the wild. Mostly raw meat, bones, maybe some feathers and fur. The only grain they would eat would be the tiny amount of fermented grains that were in the stomach contents of their prey. And grains are very aging.

Of course you may not be able to match this diet, but we have anthropomorphised our pets to such a degree that we think we want to 'humanise' their food. Delicacies. Constant variety. Not to mention continuous nibbling and treats. The sad fact is that we are killing them with kindness.

Dried kibble is bad news, especially to cats. In nature, cats rarely drink. They get all the liquid they need from the blood of their prey. A cat's kidneys are designed to process only tiny amounts of fluid. But when they eat dried food they have to drink much more. After years of this their kidneys are shot and all sorts of infections and diseases become common.

The 'snacking' trend is not healthy either. When an animal smells food, digestive hormones are activated. Other activities, like regeneration and assimilation, are temporarily suspended while the body focuses on eating. Then after eating the body switches off these hormones as they assimilate. Other processes, like regeneration and healing, are activated. This is the feast and famine flow of nature. When your cat has a twenty-four/seven access to food, these vital processes are messed with. The digestive hormones are chronically stimulated. This creates an environment for degenerative diseases to flourish.

I am not telling you what to do. I have no degree in veterinarian science. I know I want my pets to live healthy pain-free lives as much as is possible. I like to use my vets, like my doctors, only for injuries and accidents. Not chronic disease caused by the food industry.

CHAPTER 25

◆—◆—◆

Things to Avoid

Aspartame

If it says 'sugar-free' then avoid it like the plague. Sugar-free usually means it is made with the neuro-toxin, aspartame. Known as 'Nutra-sweet', 'Sweet 'n Low', 'Equal' and so on. It is added to pretty much all 'diet' drinks and foods. Banned in many countries around the world, *we* still think it is okay to consume. MS, Alzheimer's, arthritis, chronic fatigue, Parkinson's, and panic disorders are just some diseases which are made worse by this neuro-toxin. It is found everywhere these days. Breath mints, chewing gum, yoghurt, vitamins, medicines, baby formula, shake mixes. It depletes serotonin (you know, the feel-good hormone) and doesn't even help you to lose weight.

You have been warned!

Soy

The anti-nutrient passed off as a health product. Do the tiniest bit of research and you will see that this phytoestrogen should not be consumed in any quantity, and traditionally never was. Customarily in Asian cuisine, it was fermented and used as a condiment only.

The health food industry juggernaut has taken it on in typical overzealous fashion. Hundreds of thousands of hectares are given over to its production. It is forced, often unknowingly, down our throats. It is in pretty much *all* processed foods. Take a look at the tiny six-point type that is the ingredient list and in most processed foods you will find it there. Known by many names including; soy, soya, soya bean, lecithin, TVP, hydrolysed plant protein, guar, xanthan, HSP, natural flavouring to name just a few.

It is everywhere and it is wreaking havoc on our health. Our hormone system. Our nutritional assimilation. Our allergic reactions. Many auto-immune and mystery illness can lay their origins at the feet of this one.

Start reading the ingredients list, if you can see it, and avoid where possible. Or better still follow my next tip...

Processed anything

Here's a little game I like to play. It's called: imagine how they made this? I have a slightly jaded view of the food processing industry. I know the picture on the label, you know, of a country kitchen complete with red checked table cloth and green hills out the window, is not where this came from. I know that jam/chutney/bread/sauce/dressing has never seen a kitchen like that. But what is the reality? What *does* a yoghurt making factory look like? Smell like? Just how many listed and unlisted chemicals *are* they adding?

The food manufacturing industry is a behemoth. Faceless, nameless bottom-line creature. That mouldy produce *you* would throw out make it in to production. After all, it's only a few in a vat the size of your house being boiled up to temperatures that destroy all traces of mould. And vitamins. And pretty much everything of value.

The cancer causing (or the 'jury's still out' or 'it hasn't even been tested') chemical that is being added to give shine, silky texture, consistency or taste (because the taste has been 'pasteurized' out in those giant boiling vats) is only one in one hundred thousand parts, so really, it is no worse than breathing fumes or smoking a cigarette. So what the big deal?

Become informed so you can make a choice. An informed, intelligent choice. Don't plead ignorance when you have chronic insidious health issues like headaches, fatigue or menstrual pain. When your children develop behavioural issues. Or asthma. Or worse. Get smart. Get informed. Then take action.

Or not. That is up to you.

Sugar

Do I have to? There is enough written these days on the subject that I am sure you know the dangers of this particular addiction.

Gluten

Most of us do better without it. Or with very little. It seems to induce a brain fog as well as the digestive imbalance. The problem is, like sugar and caffeine, it is ubiquitous. There is probably not a day that you go without it. So you have no base line. No way of knowing what it feels like *without* 'gluten-brain'.

The only way is to eliminate it totally for a minimum of three weeks. And I meant totally. Not even a whiff. It is hard but not impossible! See how you feel after three weeks. Then re-introduce it back into your diet in tiny quantities. And note any reactions. Physical as well as emotional. Tired? Bloated? Wind? Just get to know your body and what works, or does not, for you.

Fluoride

There are some things we have a choice in and others that are chosen for us. For many countries exposure to fluoride falls into the latter category. There are so many studies done now on the destructive nature of fluoride that it is ludicrous, bordering on criminal, that it is force fed to the masses via the public water system. Reverse osmosis filtration is the only way to effectively remove it. Avoid if possible but if not, the best antidote to fluoride is iodine, as already discussed.

Antibacterial anything

It seems to be the thing, to slap an anti-bacterial label on all sorts of products. This plays into our fear of the 'unknown'. You know those invisible nasties; germs that make us sick and give our children diseases. But, what if the real nasties were the anti-bacterial itself?

We have lived with 'germs' for ever. Our immune systems have developed alongside them. Their absence actually weakens our immune system. But worse. Antibacterial substances directly and negativity affect the thyroid. Now they don't put that in the ads with the smiling, germ-free family, do they? The same receptor sites on your thyroid that absorb iodine and make it work properly, are taken up by these products. So even if you do get some iodine in your diet, if you have bought into the antibacterial brigade and have been continuously exposed to the all manner of soaps and washes and hand wipes and bench wipes and sprays and creams, your thyroid will not actually be able to absorb it.

What are the early symptoms of an underactive thyroid? Fatigue. Weight gain. Hair loss. Constipation. Memory weakness. Depression. Joint pain.

So no, it may not be old age at all. It may be those nasty hand wipes you've been using.

Chemical anything

Shampoo. Soap. Washing powder. Dishwashing liquid, Sunscreen. Moisturizer. Insect repellent. Deodorant. Tooth paste. Water bottles. Plastic wrap. The list is endless. We are swimming in a chemical cocktail. The cure for cancer is not in a laboratory filled with rats, funded by charity and government grants. C'mon do you trust Mr. Bayer, Roche, Pfizer, or Johnston with your future? Do they really care about your health as deeply as you do? Might they have an agenda when they offer to jab, pop, smear or inhale the latest and greatest wonder-drug? Just get informed. Do your research. And be proactive. There are alternatives to everything. Alternatives that some major company is not making a profit from.

Mind state

By far, the most destructive thing you can do for your health is hold a disturbed mind state. If any of the above makes you mad, makes you sad or disturbs you, you are just adding to the trouble.

Your thoughts are real forces. A thought creates an emotional reaction. An emotional reaction causes hormonal changes. Think of how you feel when you are furious. Or in love. Or excited. These all have corresponding hormones and chemicals that are released into the blood stream and that your cells are bathed in. What do you think a constant bath of 'anger' will do to the health of your internal organs? Or sadness? Or indignation? It will cause more damage than any amount of fluoride or chemicals will.

And the good news is, if you are exposed to the one, at least you have a choice about the other. That does not mean you become passive or inactive. But you can take positive action without disrupting your mind. You can make changes without losing your cool.

See chapter twenty-one on meditation to start the process on getting to know your mind and how to master it.

CHAPTER 26

Confession

Okay, here goes! The real goal of this book is to bring you to a more confident, more connected, more empowered you. There is nothing as sexy as a confident woman who *knows* she is sexy. No matter her age or her outer appearance. I guarantee that air of confidence will do more to make you attractive than one-hundred thousand dollars of plastic surgery ever will.

Care for your body. Respect and nurture it. You only get one. But more importantly respect and care for your inner self. What your mind thinks will show up on your face. If you love and accept yourself, you will have a face of beauty. If you hate and resent yourself, your aging, you will have a face of stress.

The choice is yours and you make it a million times every day.

Note on Index of Ailments

I have to say this as no doubt some will see 'Cancer' or 'High Blood Pressure' on the list and assume I am trying to replace your doctor or your own common sense. *I am not.* Your health is a dynamic and elusive beast that you alone are responsible for. If you suffer from any of the following ailments then I sincerely hope you are being completely proactive. This list (and book) should be seen as but a tool in your arsenal to fight not only aging, but the many aspects of disease. That means *not* leaving it up to me, to your doctor or to fate to take charge and 'fix' the situation.

My strong suggestion is that you explore every avenue available to realise full health. Some of these techniques may not work for you – well, then don't use them! Although I am a health professional, I would never presume to prescribe without a consultation. Even then, I always advise my patent listen to what *their* body is telling them. Having said that, all of the following are what is generally known as 'food therapy' or 'lifestyle changes' that lead to sustainable and complete illness reversal. There are rarely any adverse side effects. And there is certainly no agenda. No one is getting rich selling lemons. Or kale.

My attitude to health is to be as proactive as possible, to try and test and experiment. Be your own double blind test and see what works. Listen to your body. Learn. And the best part? None of these techniques have negative side effects an all have positive side benefits. So if imposing a 'News Embargo' does not help your anxiety – at least you have not lost anything, spent anything or developed a nasty addiction in the process. And in the long term you may find that it does increase happiness. None of these are a quick fix – so you need to get out of the take a pill and it's all better mindset. These are lifestyle changes. It took a decade to create your digestive imbalance (you probably ignored the tiny warning signs for years) so don't think it can be cured overnight. Or in a week. These change are recommended as lifestyle adjustments. But apply the 80/20 rule. If you implement 20% of these techniques 80% of the time you are without a doubt going to be a whole heap better off.

At the end of the day, you need to take responsibility for *your* body. When it comes to *your* body *you* are the expert and everyone else (including me) is simply an advisor.

Index of Ailments

Acne ....1 Lemon Drench

....11 Green Smoothie

Acidity ....1 Lemon Drench

....11 Green Smoothie

Adrenals ....11 Green Smoothie

....13 Earthing

....17 News Embargo

....18 Sleep Dark

.... 21 Meditation

Allergies ....1 Lemon Drench

.... 3 Body Brush

....11 Green Smoothie

.... 12 Deep Breathing

Anaemia ....11 Green Smoothie

.... 25 Fluoride/Processed Anything

Anxiety ....11 Green Smoothie

....13 Earthing

.... 17 News Embargo

....18 Sleep Dark

.... 21 Meditation

.... 25 Aspartame

Atherosclerosis.................................... 1 Lemon Drench

.... 3 Body Brush

....8 Stretching

.... 11 Green Smoothie

.... 24 Salt

....25 Sugar/Processed Anything

Arthritis .... 1 Lemon Drench

.... 3 Body Brush

....8 Stretching

.... 10 Sunning

....13 Earthing

.... 24 Salt

Asthma.. 2 Hot/Cold Therapy

.... 12 Deep Breathing

....25 Soy/Gluten

.... 26 Chemical anything

Bad Breath.. 1 Lemon Drench

.... 3 Body Brush

....7 Oil Pulling

11 Green Smoothie

12 Deep Breathing

15 Perfect Poo

Blood Pressure, high 1 Lemon Drench

2 Hot Cold Therapy

11 Green Smoothie

8 Stretching

12 Deep Breathing

21 Meditation

24 Salt

25 Aspartame

Blood Pressure, low 2 Hot/Cold Therapy

3 Body Brush

11 Green Smoothie

13 Earthing

18 Sleep Dark

24 Salt

25 Sugar/Fluoride

Body Odour 1 Lemon Drench

3 Body Brush

7 Oil Pulling

11 Green Smoothie

14 Salt Brine

....15 Perfect Poo

....25 Processed Anything

Bone Health ....8 Stretch

....10 Sunning

....11 Green Smoothies

....25 Soy/Gluten/Antibacterial

Bowel Disorders ....1 Lemon Drench

....11 Green Smoothie

....15 Perfect Poo

....16 Yoni Bath

....19 Food Blessing

....23 Attitude

....24 Lugol's

....25 Gluten/Processed Anything

Brain Health ....3 Body Brush

....6 Eye Exercises

....10 Sunning

....11 Green Smoothie

....15 Perfect Poo

....17 News Embargo

....18 Sleep Dark

....19 Food Blessing

....23 Attitude

.............................25 Gluten/Processed/Chemical Anything

Cancer .... 3 Body Brush

.... 4 Face Gym

....7 Oil Pulling

.... 9 Journaling

.... 10 Sunning

....11 Green Smoothie

....13 Earthing

.... 15 Perfect Poo

....18 Sleep Dark

....21 Meditation

.... 25 All in this chapter

Cellulite ....1 Lemon Drench

.... 3 Body Brush

.... 12 Deep Breathing

.... 15 Perfect Poo

....24 Lugol's

.............................25 Antibacterial/Chemical Anything

Cholesterol ....1 Lemon Drench

....11 Green Smoothie

.............................25 Antibacterial Anything/Fluoride

Chronic Fatigue .... 9 Journaling

.... 10 Sunning

.... 11 Green Smoothie

.... 12 Deep Breathing

....13 Earthing

....15 Perfect Poo

.... 17 News Embargo

....18 Sleep Dark

....24 Lugol's

.... 25 All in this chapter

Circulation Problems .... 2 Hot/Cold Therapy

.... 3 Body Brush

....8 Stretch

.... 12 Deep Breathing

....13 Earthing

....24 Lugol's

.... 25 Processed Anything

Colds & Flu .... 1 Lemon Drench

....7 Oil Pulling

.... 10 Sunning

.... 11 Green Smoothie

....13 Earthing

.... 17 News Embargo

....18 Sleep Dark

....25 Sugar/Processed Anything

Constipation ....1 Lemon Drench
.... 3 Body Brush
........8 Stretch
.... 9 Journaling
........11 Green Smoothie
.... 15 Perfect Poo
........25 Gluten

Depression .... 9 Journaling
.... 10 Sunning
........11 Green Smoothie
........17 News Embargo
........18 Sleep Dark
.... 19 Food Blessing
........20 Insect
........21 Meditation
.... 23 Attitude
........24 Lugol's
.... 25 All in this chapter

Digestive Issues ....1 Lemon Drench
.... 3 Body Brush
........11 Green Smoothie
.... 15 Perfect Poo
.... 19 Food Blessing

....24 Lugol's

.......................25 Processed Anything/Gluten/Soy

Gout.. 1 Lemon Drench

.... 3 Body Brush

.... 10 Sunning

.... 11 Green Smoothie

.... 25 Soy/Aspartame

Headaches .... 1 Lemon Drench

....3 Body Brush

.... 4 Face Gym

....5 Face Massage

....6 Eye Exercises

.... 9 Journaling

.... 10 Sunning

.... 11 Green Smoothie

....15 Perfect Poo

.... 17 News Embargo

....18 Sleep Dark

....24 Lugol's

.... 25 All in this chapter

Infertility ....13 Earthing

.... 16 Yoni Bath

.... 25 All in this chapter

Kidney ....1 Lemon Drench

....11 Green Smoothie

....24 Salt

.... 25 Fluoride

Liver ....1 Lemon Drench

.... 3 Body Brush

.... 15 Perfect Poo

....17 News Embargo

....21 Meditation

.... 25 Chemical Anything

Lung Issues .... 2 Hot/Cold Therapy

.... 3 Body Brush

....5 Face Massage

....7 Oil Pulling

.... 9 Journaling

.... 10 Sunning

.... 12 Deep Breathing

....17 News Embargo

.... 23 Attitude

.... 25 Chemical Anything

Memory .... 3 Body Brush

....5 Face Massage

.... 10 Sunning

.... 11 Green Smoothie

.... 12 Deep Breathing

.... 21 Meditation

.... 25 Fluoride/Gluten

Menopause .... 2 Hot/Cold Therapy

.... 3 Body Brush

.... 9 Journaling

.... 10 Sunning

.... 11 Green Smoothie

.... 12 Deep Breathing

.... 16 Yoni Bath

.... 25 Gluten

Menstrual Irregularities .... 3 Body brush

.... 9 Journaling

.... 11 Green Smoothie

.... 16 Yoni Bath

.... 25 Soy

Pancreas .... 1 Lemon Drench

.... 3 Body Brush

.... 10 Sunning

.... 11 Green Smoothie

.... 12 Earthing

.... 15 Perfect Poo

.... 25 Sugar/Fluoride

Pet Ailments ....24 Pet diet

Skin problems ....1 Lemon Drench

.... 2 Hot/Cold Therapy

.... 3 Body Brush

....11 Green Smoothie

.... 12 Deep Breathing

.... 15 Perfect Poo

....25 Sugar

Sleep Problems .... 8 Stretch

.... 9 Journaling

.... 10 Sunning

....11 Green Smoothie

.... 12 Deep Breathing

....13 Earthing

....17 News Embargo

....18 Sleep Dark

....21 Meditation

Teeth problems ....7 Oil Pulling

....5 Face Massage

....11 Green Smoothie

.... 19 Food Blessing

Thyroid ....1 Lemon Drench

.... 10 Sunning

.... 11 Green Smoothie

.... 12 Deep Breathing

....15 Perfect Poo

....18 Sleep Dark

....24 Lugol's

.... 25 Soy/Fluoride/Antibacterial Anything

Tiredness ....10 Sunning

.... 11 Green Smoothie

.... 12 Deep Breathing

....13 Earthing

....15 Perfect Poo

.... 17 News Embargo

....18 Sleep Dark

....24 Lugol's

.............................25 Gluten/Sugar/Processed Anything

Toxicity .... 1 Lemon Drench

.... 2 Hot/Cold Therapy

.... 3 Body Brush

....5 Face Massage

....7 Oil Pulling

.... 9 Journaling

....10 Sunning

....11 Green Smoothie

.... 12 Deep Breathing

....15 Perfect Poo

....16 Yoni Bath

....17 News Embargo

.... 19 Food Blessing

....21 Meditation

.... 23 Attitude

.... 25 All in this chapter

Urinary infections ....1 Lemon Drench

.... 9 Journaling

....11 Green Smoothie

....16 Yoni Bath

Vision problems ....5 Face Massage

.... 6 Eye Exercises

.... 10 Sunning

....11 Green Smoothie

....18 Sleep Dark

Weight Gain ....1 Lemon Drench

....11 Green Smoothie

....15 Perfect Poo

....18 Sleep Dark

.... 23 Attitude

....24 Lugol's

....25 Aspartame/Sugar

....................................25 Antibacterial/Processed Anything

Facial Wrinkles .... 3 Body Brush

.... 4 Face Gym

....5 Face Massage

....6 Eye Exercises

.... 9 Journaling

.... 17 News Embargo

.... 21 Meditation

....24 Lugol's

.... 25 Gluten/Fluoride/Processed Anything

A gift for you...
Infographic of the Book

Go to https://app.convertkit.com/landing_pages/81870?v=6 to grab your free infographic – a visual representation of every technique in the book for you to print out and hang on the wall as a visual reminder.

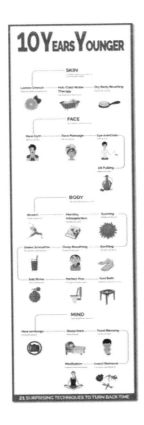

About the Author

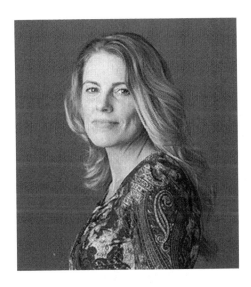

After growing up without electricity, running water and several hours from the nearest shops Kylie Ansett knows a thing or two about 'roughing it'. At that time books and a vivid imagination were her only source of entertainment. Both reading and writing she soon learned the power of the written word.

Her other passions include teaching, health & healing and coaching. After both Kylie's books became #1 Amazon best sellers, she now teaches others the art & science of creating & marketing a successful book.

These days she lives in Sydney, Australia, where she enjoys the exhilarating, tenuous and always stimulating life of an entrepreneur: writing, coaching, training and creating.

Other Books by Kylie:
Bodyworker's Success Blueprint

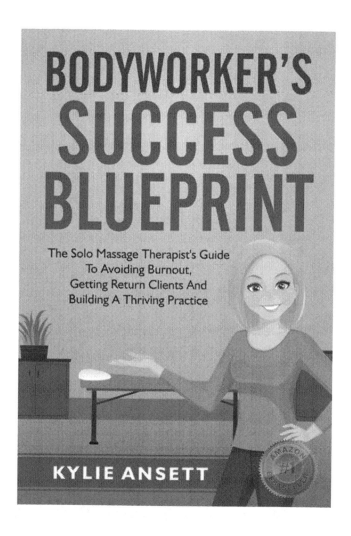

Bodyworker's Success Blueprint

Take Control of Your Business & Build the Practice of Your Dreams. Is it possible to make a living, a good living, with your two hands? Do you dream of having a successful massage business? Do you wish for more clients on your table and more dollars in your wallet? Do you wonder if you can keep doing this work long-term? Can you avoid bodyworker burnout?

This book is for people who are serious about building a successful massage or therapy practice. Packed with empowering techniques to get your dream career off to a great start, simple strategies to grow a vibrant practice and effective ideas to support your clients in their healing journey – all without sacrificing your own health along the way.

Most of us dream of success but we don't always know where to start to make those dreams a reality. In her 15 years as a therapist, Kylie has seen it all. She learned the hard way how to manage her energy and her mind to achieve the success she yearned for.

Bodyworker's Success Blueprint is practical, actionable and just a bit irreverent. You will both laugh and learn as you read.

Book Writing & Marketing Courses by Kylie:

Book Launch Boot Camp

I thought *writing* the book was the hard part... After hitting publish I soon discovered there is a whole world of hustle, publicity and promotions to get on with – otherwise your book sinks to the bottom of the Amazon quicksand never to be seen or heard from again.

Book Launch Boot Camp is your guiding light to negotiate the tricky path to bestseller success. From the science of marketing persuasion to the Amazon rankings game – this course covers it all.

Go to www.booklaunchbootcamp.com

Skill2Book

From blank page to bestseller - the step by step process to take you from the burning desire to write a book – but no idea where to start or even what to write it on, through the process of writing your masterpiece, right through to becoming a published bestselling author with a work to be proud of.

Whether authoring a book would grow your current business, give you prestige and authority in your field, or simply satisfy an inner desire to share you knowledge, Skill2Book will take your lifetime of skills and talents and show you the simple, actionable process to turn them into a book that will benefit many.

Go to: www.Skill2book.com

Made in the USA
San Bernardino, CA
07 February 2017